Contents

Preface

• Hair and scalp disorders are more frequently encountered in medical practice than might be imagined. They encompass, on the whole, a number of conditions which, while they are not life threatening, nevertheless are of very great concern to the patient or their parents. The management of these conditions is frequently an intellectual challenge not necessarily in diagnosis but long-term management, from neonatal 'cradle cap' to severe and continual hair loss.

• It is unsatisfactory to dismiss patients with suggestions of triviality. Physicians will be required to occasionally manage complex and difficult cases of hair loss where patient expectations of cure are as high as for more serious diseases. Sadly, the doctor's armamentarium is currently bare.

• The successful management of cases epitomizes both the art and the science of medicine.

• This book has been produced to provide a visual guide to diagnosis and assist in the management of some of the more common disorders.

• For a more comprehensive treatment of the subject, R. Dawber: *Diseases of the Hair and Scalp*, Blackwell Science, 1997 is recommended.

• We hope this book will be of value to medical students, practising physicians and healthcare workers.

Acknowledgements

We would like to thank the following people for providing photographs: Dr David Whiting, Dr Ron Savin and Dr Dominique Van Neste. We would also like to thank Janet Smith for her patient organization and coordination of this project.

Finally, we would both like to thank our respective families for their understanding during the writing of this book.

John Gray
Rodney Dawber
July 1998

A Pocketbook of

Hair and Scalp Disorders

An

EDHCC

10010769

Joh

MBBᵤ, ...,
General Practitioner and Medical Consultant P&G (Europe)
Procter & Gamble
Lovett House
Lovett Road
S....

Books are to be returned on or before
the last date below.

www.librex.co.uk

© 1999 by
Blackwell Science Ltd
Editorial Offices:
Osney Mead, Oxford OX2 oEL
25 John Street, London WC1N 2BL
23 Ainslie Place, Edinburgh EH3
    6AJ
350 Main Street, Malden
    MA 02148 5018, USA
54 University Street, Carlton
    Victoria 3053, Australia
10, rue Casimir Delavigne
    75006 Paris, France

Other Editorial Offices:
Blackwell Wissenschafts-Verlag
    GmbH
Kurfürstendamm 57
10707 Berlin, Germany

Blackwell Science KK
MG Kodenmacho Building
7–10 Kodenmacho Nihombashi
Chuo-ku, Tokyo 104, Japan

The right of the Authors to be
identified as the Authors of this
Work has been asserted in
accordance with the copyright,
Designs and Patents Act 1988.

First published 1999

Set by Excel Typesetters Co.,
Hong Kong

The Blackwell Science logo
is a trade mark of Blackwell
Science Ltd, registered at
the United Kingdom
Trade Marks Registry

DISTRIBUTORS

Marston Book Services Ltd
PO Box 269,
Abingdon, Oxon OX14 4YN
(*Orders*: Tel: 01235 465500
            Fax: 01235 465555)

USA
Blackwell Science, Inc.
Commerce Place
350 Main Street
Malden, MA 02148 5018
(*Orders*: Tel: 800 759 6102
                  781 388 8250
           Fax: 781 388 8255)

Canada
Login Brothers Book Company
324 Saulteaux Cresent
Winnipeg, Manitoba R3J 3T2
(*Orders*: Tel: 204 837-2987)

Australia
Blackwell Science Pty Ltd
54 University Street
Carlton, Victoria 3053
(*Orders*: Tel: 3 9347 0300
           Fax: 3 9347 5001)

A catalogue record for this title
is available from the British Library

ISBN 0-632-05189-2

Library of Congress
Cataloging-in-publication Data

Gray, John, 1947 Nov. 25–
    A pocketbook of hair and
    scalp disorders: an illustrated
    guide/John Gray, Rodney
    Dawber.
        p.   cm.
    ISBN 0-632-05189-2
    1. Hair–Diseases–Handbooks,
    manuals, etc.   2. Scalp–
    Diseases–Handbooks, manuals,
    etc. I. Dawber, R.P.R. (Rodney
    P.R.) II. Title.
        [DNLM: 1. Hair Diseases
    handbooks.   2. Scalp
    handbooks.   3. Skin Diseases
    handbooks. WR 39G779p
    1998]
    RL 151.G73   1998
    616.5′46–dc21
    DNLM/DLC
    for Library of Congress
                            98-26852
                                CIP

For further information on
Blackwell Science, visit our website:
www.blackwell-science.com

1: Hair structure, physiology and properties

Types of hair

Three distinct types of hair grow on the human body.

LANUGO HAIR

This is the hair that develops on the fetus after about the 20th week of the pregnancy. The hairs grow uniformly and synchronously, as in moulting animals. At around the 36th week these hairs are shed *in utero*. If a fetus is born prematurely, it may still be covered in this 'down'.

At normal gestation the infant has two types of hair: 'vellus hair' and 'terminal hair'.

VELLUS HAIR

Vellus hairs are fine, short (1–2 cm) hairs, containing little or no pigment and growing from hair follicles with no sebaceous glands (Fig. 1.1). These follicles can only produce vellus hairs.

TERMINAL HAIR

Terminal hairs are the 'normal' long, thick hairs that grow on the scalp, face, chest and arms before puberty; after puberty they also grow at secondary hair sites i.e. on the axillae, arms and legs. These grow from follicles that have sebaceous glands. In conditions such as male and female pattern baldness, hairs in these so-called 'terminal follicles' can gradually become thinner and shorter to mimic vellus hairs.

Variations with age

CHILDHOOD

At birth, terminal hairs are found only in the scalp, eyebrows and eyelashes. Vellus hairs are present elsewhere on the body. After birth two waves of hair develop on the head, growing over the scalp from the forehead to the nape of the neck. There is an area on the back of the head where all the hairs may be shed naturally at 8–12

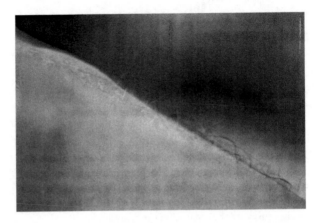

Fig. 1.1 Vellus hairs exist at all sites except soles and palms.

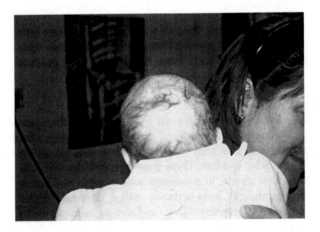

Fig. 1.2 An area of alopecia due to shedding of hair at 8–12 weeks. This is a normal phenomenon.

weeks. This is often wrongly attributed to head rubbing (Fig. 1.2) but it can be a normal physiological process; unlike rubbing or pressure, this is not accompanied by hair breakage.

Immediately after birth the hairs on the head grow at the same rate, and the hair appears to grow in an even pattern.

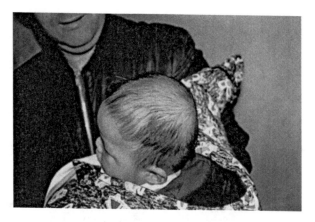

Fig. 1.3 Mosaic patterns develop at the end of the first year as hairs begin to grow asynchronously.

At the end of the first year of life, the individual hairs begin to grow in their own separate cycles and terminal hair growth becomes asynchronous, such that a mosaic of hair growth develops (Fig. 1.3).

ADOLESCENCE

From birth onwards, the scalp carries a mixture of many long terminal hairs and some short vellus hairs. After puberty in both sexes many of the hairs on the limbs and trunk change to terminal hairs, the so-called postpubertal, secondary 'sexual' hair. The hair shaft becomes thicker and longer. In males, many terminal hairs develop on the beard area on the face and neck under the influence of androgens.

MIDDLE AGE AND BEYOND

With ageing, scalp hair can still grow strongly but the period during which the hairs grow actively tends to shorten, and hairs tend to become shorter and thinner, particularly on the crown. Some site specificity develops; in men this results in strong growth of terminal hairs in predetermined androgen-dependent sites (the nose, ears and eyebrows) well into old age, as hair growth tends to decline on the top of the head (Fig. 1.4).

Grey hairs tend to be coarser and often medullated. They

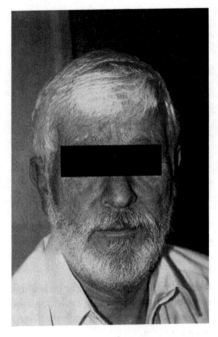

Fig. 1.4 Androgen-dependent sites: bitemporal recession, bushy eyebrows and beard, associated with almost total loss of pigment.

seem to be more resistant to the patchy hair loss associated with alopecia areata (see Chapter 2).

The structure of a hair

The scalp hair follicle
Hair is technically dead, yet a single hair can grow for years.

The human scalp has some 100 000–150 000 hair follicles (the number has been determined embryologically). The density of the follicles decreases with age, from about 500–700 per cm² at birth to 250–350 per cm² as an adult as the scalp area increases.

Each follicle (Fig. 1.5) grows a hair continuously for between 2 and 7 years, potentially producing a terminal hair in excess of 1 m in length (Fig. 1.6).

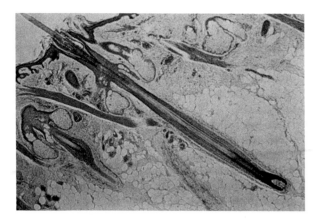

Fig. 1.5 Histological section of the hair follicle in anagen. The hair bulb is buried deep in the subcutaneous fat.

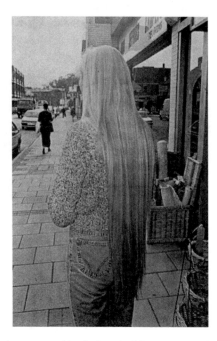

Fig. 1.6 As we grow older the length of the active growth phase (anagen) tends to decrease. This lady has retained her ability for prolonged anagen well into her fifth decade.

Each scalp follicle on average grows 20–30 hairs in a lifetime.

The hair follicle is situated during active growth in, or just above, the subcutaneous fat at core temperature. It is protected from any deleterious effects of materials on the scalp. Only severe scarring or systemic factors interfere with hair growth.

The hair follicle is divided anatomically into the:
- **infundibulum;**
- **isthmus;** and
- **inferior segment,** which contains the **hair bulb.**

About 95% of the follicles on the scalp are in an active growth phase (anagen, see Chapter 2).

The hair root

Hair is actively and continuously generated in the hair bulb from the **matrix.** This consists of actively dividing cells enveloping the **dermal papilla;** these are the mesenchymal cells that orchestrate the cyclical growth (Fig. 1.7).

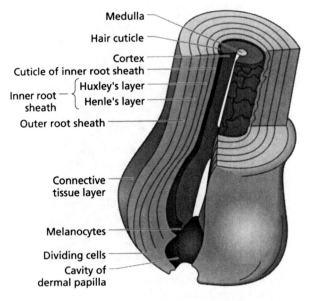

Fig. 1.7 Diagrammatic representation of the hair bulb.

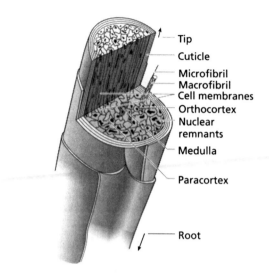

Fig. 1.8 Diagrammatic representation of the hair shaft.

The hair shaft (Fig. 1.8)
Rapidly dividing cells are forced upwards and differentiate into areas which form the hair shaft; these are the:
• cortical cells;
• inner root sheath; and
• outer root sheath.
Cortical cells are denucleated derivatives of medullary cells. They produce protein fibrils, which become increasingly compacted into macro fibrils; these are enmeshed in an amorphous matrix rich in sulphydryl groups. This increasingly keratinized cortex bestows most of the physical properties, including volume and strength, of the hair shaft. Some hairs, particularly those which are unpigmented, have a central air space, the **medulla** (a feature which is of no great importance in humans). An outer casing, the **cuticle**, develops from the root sheath. The cuticle is 6–10 cells thick; the cells are regularly spaced at intervals of 10 μm, overlapping from root to tip of the hair shaft (Fig. 1.9).

Physical characteristics of hair
The **shape** (Fig. 1.10) of an individual's hair is genetically determined. The inner and outer root sheaths assist in

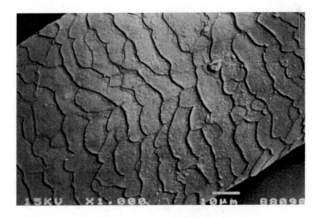

Fig. 1.9 EMG of a normal hair shaft, showing the regular 10 μm repeat of the cuticular cells.

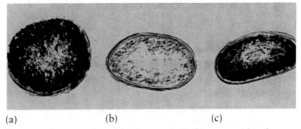

(a)   (b)   (c)

Fig. 1.10 Cross-sections of (a) mongoloid, (b) caucasoid and (c) negroid hair, showing the morphological differences.

moulding the keratinizing cortex cells, and the basic shape of the individual hair is determined by:
- the shape of the follicular outlet;
- the position of the hair bulb within the follicle; and
- any irregularities of mitosis within the hair bulb.

There are three basic hair shapes, which are related to the major racial types:
- Mongoloid (Oriental);
- Caucasoid (European and Indian); and
- Negroid (African).

Negroid hair is distinctly more ovoid in cross-section than are the other types. This confers a greater vulnerability to damage, particularly heat and physical damage.

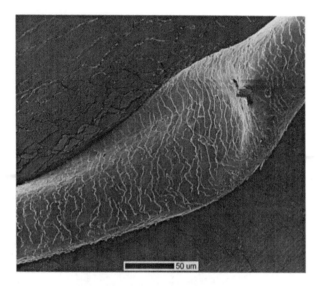

Fig. 1.11 Negroid hair, showing severe distortion from twisting.

A considerable degree of polymorphism has occurred over many centuries, with the consequent appearance of mixed characteristics, particularly among the Caucasian peoples and in countries with a history of very significant immigration (such as the UK and USA).

Hair **diameter** varies between 50 μm (typical of Caucasian, particularly Nordic, hair) and 120 μm (Asiatic hair).

Hair **twist** characteristics are also genetically predetermined. Even apparently straight hair twists. Negroid hair twists some 12 times more frequently per unit length than does Caucasian hair (Fig. 1.11).

Hair colour

Hair colour is determined by the presence of melanin granules derived from melanocytes in the hair medulla (Fig. 1.12).

There are two fundamental types of melanin:

• eumelanin (brown); and

9

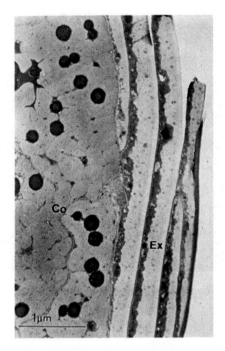

Fig. 1.12 Melanin granules distributed along the cortex of the hair shaft.

• phaeomelanin (blonde/red, especially common in Celtic races).

Different combinations of melanins produce differing shades of colour.

The most common hair colour in the world is black.

GREYING OF HAIR

Grey hair is a reflection of ageing and is due to a progressive reduction in melanin production.

There is a gradual dilution of pigment in greying hairs. A full range of colour from normal to white can be seen along individual hairs and from hair to hair. The age at which greying begins is again dependent on genetic factors.

In Caucasian races, 50% of the population have at least 50% of grey hairs on the scalp at the age of 50. The temples usually show greying first, followed by a wave of greyness spreading first from the crown and then to the back.

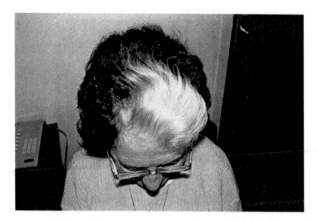

Fig. 1.13 Silver hair, developed at about age 16, inherited from mother/grandmother.

Premature greying

Premature greying can begin before 20 years of age in Caucasians and 30 years of age in Negroids, though it normally has little visual impact at this age. It probably has (again) a genetic basis (Fig. 1.13).

How many hairs do we have?
- On *average*, each of us has about 100 000 hair follicles on our head. In some people the number may be as high as 150 000.
- The average density of hair follicles on an infant head is 500–700 per cm².
- This density progressively decreases as the head enlarges during childhood and adolescence, such that in adult life this number falls to 250–350 per cm². There is only a slight further reduction in old age.
- Each of these follicles may grow 20–30 new hairs in a lifetime.
- Each new hair can grow for between 2 and 7 years and reach more than 1 m in length before it enters a resting period lasting about 3 months when it is shed.

Continued on p. 12

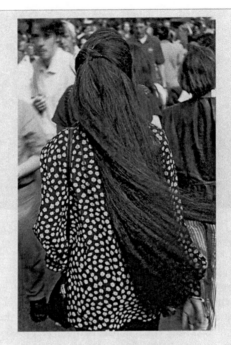

Fig. 1.14

- As a rule 95% of scalp hairs are growing actively and 5% are in a resting phase.
- As we grow older the time the hair will actively grow tends to decrease and our hair naturally is shorter.
- Each resting hair will eventually fall out to be replaced by a new growing one.

2: Hair loss

Hair loss, or alopecia (the term is derived from the Greek word *alopekia*, signifying a fox—a species that suffers from a mange-like condition), is perhaps, to the general physician, understandably of relatively low importance compared to painful or life-threatening ailments. However, the impact of real or perceived hair loss on patients should never be underestimated. In both males and females, hair loss can be psychologically devastating and socially restricting. Even slight thinning in certain 'per-morbid' personalities may lead to psychiatric symptoms, and in rare cases to suicide.

'Abnormal' hair loss as a presenting feature represents widely differing diagnoses. Hair loss, curiously, has attracted a mythology of cause and effect that is allied to 'alternative' treatments, of sometimes quite staggering absurdity.

The hair cycle
Except where there is dermal scarring, hair will continue to grow, producing a continuous keratinous structure. The 100 000–150 000 hair follicles of the scalp have at any one time some 95% in active growth phase (**anagen**), on average this lasts 1000 days. The remainder are in a resting phase (**telogen**), on average this lasts 100 days and are waiting to be shed spontaneously or removed. There is a short intervening stage (catagen) which lasts approximately 10 days. Typically hairs are shed during shampooing, combing or brushing, at a rate of 50–80 per day. If the hair is shampooed only once a week several hundred hairs may be lost simultaneously, representing the accumulated potential over several days.

This transition from anagen to catagen to telogen and return to anagen is the **hair cycle**.

It is of fundamental importance that the physician is aware of the nature of the hair cycle since it forms a basis for understanding the mechanism of abnormal loss, for

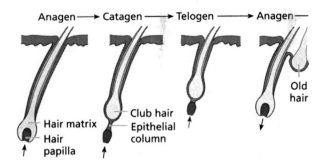

Fig. 2.1 The hair cycle.

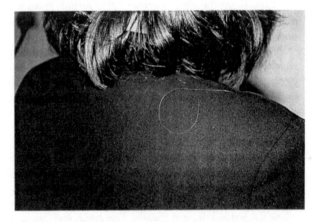

Fig. 2.2 Telogen hair seen on clothing is part of the normal everyday hair loss.

interpretation of clinical signs and for explanation to patients of the nature and prognosis of their condition.

In order to be able to discuss whether apparently excessive hair loss is 'real', an understanding of the hair cycle is necessary (Fig. 2.1).

It is telogen hairs that we see on a daily basis in the environment—in the shower, on clothing (Fig. 2.2). On occasion, however, more hairs than the average 50–80 per day *appear* to be lost. When this hair loss is significantly and persistently above average the scalp may become visible (Fig. 2.3).

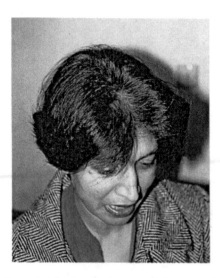

Fig. 2.3 Decreasing density of hair eventually leads to visible loss, but there may be as much as 50% reduction before this becomes apparent.

Hair density

The density of scalp hair is not constant throughout life. In extreme old age, very significant thinning may be expected. An important feature in assessing whether 'excessive' hair loss is real or perceived is an appreciation of 'anticipated hair density' and its decline with increasing age. This is of particular importance in assessing potential androgenic hair loss in females. Figure 2.4 (a and b) indicates the expected density of hair in a female and male in extreme old age.

Mechanisms of increased hair loss

The rapidly dividing matrix cells in the hair bulb may be affected by various situations in which their response can be either:
- to cease anagen prematurely, move into a resting phase (telogen) and subsequently be shed;
or
- to slow, or temporarily interrupt, the normal division and differentiation of matrix cells in anagen but upon removal of the interrupting agent, recommence anagen.

If *large* numbers of hair follicles simultaneously enter into

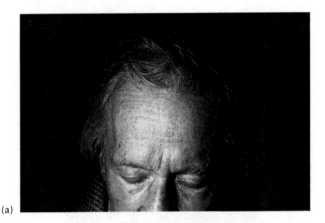

(a)

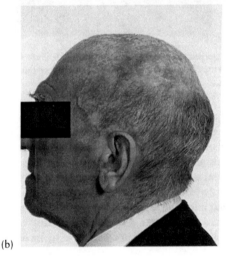

(b)

Fig. 2.4 Hair density in old age.

the resting phase (telogen), the clinical result is likely to be a **telogen effluvium**, in which significantly increased numbers of telogen hairs are seen to fall daily. Classically, telogen hair loss does not begin until 3 or 4 months after anagen ceases. Clinically the scalp will then become significantly more visible within days and weeks, depending on the number of follicles affected. Many shed telogen hairs will be visible to the naked eye.

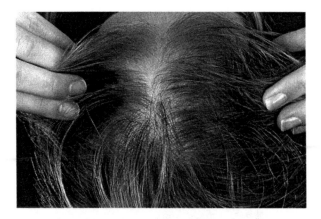

Fig. 2.5 Hair loss over many years. Gradual diffuse hair loss in women is suggestive of androgenetic alopecia.

In other conditions, this entry into telogen takes place more subtly and the clinical effects are not seen so quickly. Androgenetic alopecia is the best example of an insidious increase in the number of hairs in telogen, which can occur over many years (Fig. 2.5).

In **alopecia areata** (see below) many follicles prematurely and very rapidly enter telogen and are subsequently shed. The condition can vary from the acute (Fig. 2.6) to chronic (Fig. 2.7). The cause of the condition is unknown but this type of alopecia falls into the category of autoimmune disorders.

Interruption of **anagen production**, rather than cessation, tends to lead to a weakened hair shaft that nevertheless continues to grow. Scalp hair normally grows at the rate of 1 cm per month. Since anagen hair bulbs are located in the subcutaneous tissue ~0.4 mm from the scalp surface, it takes about 2 weeks from the time of the insult for the section of damaged anagen hair to reach the scalp surface. Once free of the supporting follicular duct, the damaged hair will generally break off at the point of the weakened shaft, producing an **anagen effluvium** (Fig. 2.8). In a patient with anagen hair breakage, the history will focus primarily on events in the **past 2–3 weeks**. This is the classical response to chemotherapy, in which virtually all the hair bulbs are affected synchronously.

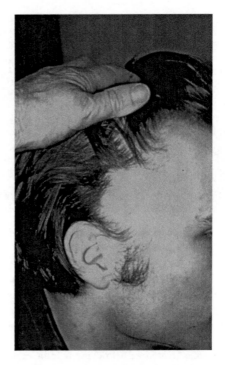

Fig. 2.6 Acute hair loss. An unusual case of acute alopecia areata, also due to an increase in telogen hair loss: these lesions were bilateral.

Differential diagnosis of hair loss

Before proceeding to the clinical aspects of management, it is worth briefly reviewing the differential morphological diagnosis of abnormal hair loss (bearing in mind the mechanisms discussed in the previous section).

Clinically, alopecias are of two principal types: **non-scarring** and **scarring**.

Non-scarring alopecias

In descending order of frequency cases of non-scarring alopecia seen in practice will most likely, but not inevitably, be:

- androgenetic alopecia (male and female);
- diffuse alopecia;
- alopecia areata;

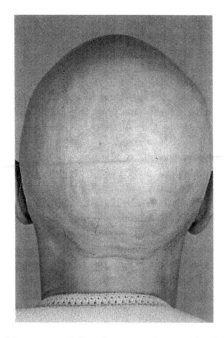

Fig. 2.7 The extreme of alopecia areata: a few surviving hairs can be seen.

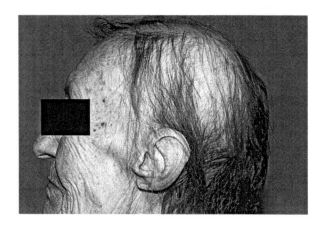

Fig. 2.8 Anagen effluvium due to chemotherapy.

- hair breakage and (rarely) loss due to cosmetic damage from physical or chemical processing;
- hair loss due to infectious conditions;
- traumatic alopecias;
- anagen effluvium;
- hair breakage and loss due to hair shaft disorders;
- loose anagen syndrome.

Each of these will be discussed in more detail in later chapters.

The most common single cause of hair loss in both sexes is certainly **androgenetic alopecia**. Patients only rarely seek medical advice. The diagnosis and lack of effective treatment can be extremely difficult for some patients to accept. Multiple opinions and 'remedies' tend to follow.

The two other commonly seen alopecias in everyday practice are **diffuse hair loss** and **alopecia areata**.

Diffuse loss is due to a range of subtle causes and is often the most difficult type of alopecia to diagnose.

Alopecia areata is often clinically obvious, and in severe forms may be dramatic for patient and doctor (Fig. 2.9).

Cosmetic damage to the hair shaft is an important cause that is often overlooked (Fig. 2.10).

Scarring alopecias

Scarring and traumatic alopecias are much less common but almost certainly occur more frequently than they are diagnosed. Scarring alopecias tend to produce permanent hair loss; they are difficult to diagnose in everyday practice and often require expert evaluation. The possible causes are many and the scarring may or may not be obvious.

In general a patchy, focal, nonpustular alopecia of the scalp is usually either lupus erythematosis (Fig. 2.11), lichen planus or pseudopelade.

Systemic lupus erythematosis (SLE) (Fig. 2.12) does not normally cause scarring alopecia but a more general telogen effluvium.

Discoid lupus erythematosis (Fig. 2.13) frequently affects the scalp, causing red, spreading lesions with central scarring.

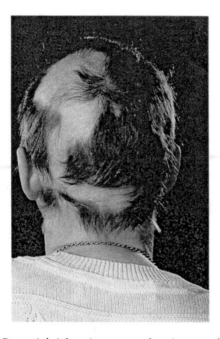

Fig. 2.9 Dramatic hair loss. Acute severe alopecia areata: the hair may be lost *en masse* when it is touched.

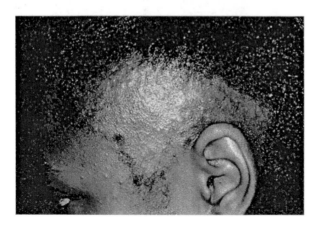

Fig. 2.10 Cosmetic damage is a common cause of apparent hair loss. Alopecia due to hair breakage as a result of oil dermatitis.

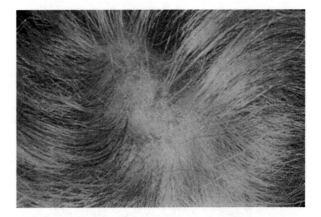

Fig. 2.11 Hair loss with scarring is associated with focal lupus erythematosis. This is the most common scarring alopecia seen in practice.

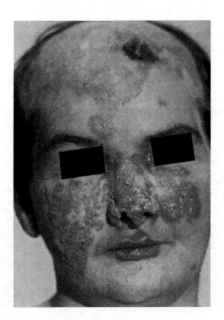

Fig. 2.12 Severe systemic lupus erythematosis. Hair loss tends to be a telogen effluvium rather than a scarring alopecia.

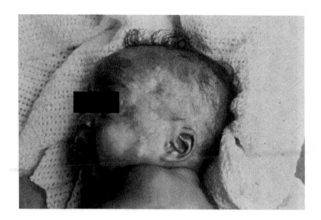

Fig. 2.13 Neonatal lupus erythematosis.

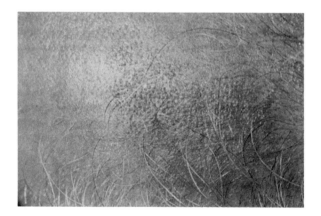

Fig. 2.14 Lichen planus.

Lichen planus (Fig. 2.14) infrequently affects the scalp, but does affect 40% of patients with unusual presentations of the disease—bullous or erosive and lichen planopilaris. Most patients are middle-aged women. Scalp lesions may show violaceous papules, erythema and scaling. Eventually scarring may occur.

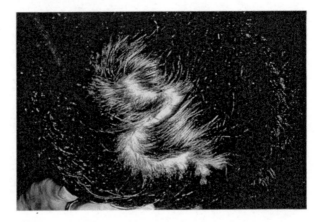

Fig. 2.15 Pseudopelade showing typical 'footstep' alopecia.

Pseudopelade (Fig. 2.15) may be a primary autoimmune atrophy of the hair follicles. It is slowly progressive, without folliculitis or inflammation. It often produces areas of triangular alopecia.

Burns are often easy to identify from the history and are usually cosmetic in origin. The possibility of chemical burns from inexpert processing (perming and dyeing) should not be forgotten; such conditions may eventually involve litigation.

Clinical assessment of hair loss
The clinical assessment of hair loss is largely a matter of common sense and practice.

The old maxim of 'history, examination and special investigations' (where appropriate) still applies. The key to diagnosis, very often, is an understanding of the implications of interruption of the hair cycle.

History
It is essential to elicit a full history in cases of perceived or obvious *recent* abnormal hair loss.

This should include a general history, particularly in cases of diffuse loss, which usually imply a general or systemic

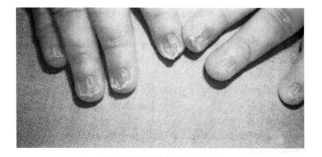

Fig. 2.16 The characteristic appearance of nails in alopecia areata. Assessment of nails may be important in diagnosis.

cause. Any history of nail disorders or familial hair disorders should be included (Fig. 2.16).

The importance of the **temporal relationship** of recent hair loss to hormonal or systemic changes cannot be emphasized enough, since this gives valuable clues as to the aetiology of the problem and leads the practitioner to give priority to investigating the organ systems potentially responsible.

A medical history in those with recent diffuse hair loss must include details of any:
• menstrual/obstetric history/childbirth;
• recent (within the previous 3 months) severe or chronic illnesses (especially thyroid, renal or hepatic disorders, or neoplasm);
• recent surgery;
• recent febrile illness;
• recent new physical complaints;
• medication within the past 6 months;
• crash dieting.

Any of these may lead to a **telogen effluvium**, since the hair bulb is susceptible to sudden changes in the internal environment.

Although hair loss may be thought of as either **acute** or **chronic** the practitioner must be alert to the inevitable continuum of one to the other. In such cases, again consider the hair cycle with hairs growing but continually entering telogen prematurely. An **acute hair loss** is likely to be an acute effluvium, alopecia areata, an infestation or an infection.

Many **chronic illnesses**, especially connective tissue disease, bowel disorders involving malabsorption, endocrine abnormalities, renal and hepatic disease and cancer (even without chemotherapy) are associated with hair loss and may be otherwise unsuspected. Certain vitamins, in particular vitamin A, can cause hair loss if taken in massive doses. Patients may not think of over-the-counter products or vitamins as medications and should be questioned specifically about their use.

In the case of **chronic hair loss** extending over 6 months or more, it is important to ascertain:
• the age at which loss became apparent (childhood, women aged 20–30 with androgenetic loss)—hair loss that begins in infancy or childhood is often of an inherited nature and may be but one component of a genetic syndrome;
• family history (androgenetic alopecia and alopecia areata);
• any relationship to hormonal changes (puberty, pregnancy, menopause, exogenous hormones).

Specific questions for the patient should include the following:
• Is the hair loss general or localized? (diffuse loss indicates a telogen effluvium, localized loss alopecia areata or infestation).
• Is the hair coming out by the roots, or breaking off? (distinguish between hair loss and hair breakage, i.e. cosmetic damage; examine the scalp with a magnifying glass).
• When did the loss start? Has it stopped? (the question relates to possible causes of the condition, such as childbirth or surgery).
• Is it continuous or intermittent? (alopecia areata (AA) may be intermittent).
• Was the loss very significant in a short time or has it been a gradual process? (AA is usually acute).
• Is the hair regrowing or is it continuing to fall?
• Is excess hair seen on comb, brush or bedding, or in the shower? (assessment of whether the daily loss is normal or abnormal).
• How often is the hair shampooed or conditioned? (assessment of daily loss).

- When was it last washed? (assessment of number of hairs lost).
- Is the hair blown dry? If yes, how often? and how hot is the dryer? (Is the problem hair breakage due to heat damage?).
- Has the hair been permed, bleached or straightened? (is the problem hair breakage due to chemical damage?).
- Are rubber bands or grips used in the hair? (is there a traction alopecia?).

The shampoo myth
Abnormal hair loss is unfortunately far too easily attributed to shampoos and conditioners by both patients and doctors, to the detriment of determining the real diagnosis.

CASE STUDIES

The following cases indicate possible pitfalls for the unwary physician.

1 A young woman presented with increased telogen hair loss three months post partum, but complained of additional patchy loss (Fig. 2.17). On examination she had evident circumscribed areas consistent with alopecia areata. She gave a positive previous history. Combined causes of alopecia are uncommon, but should not be forgotten.

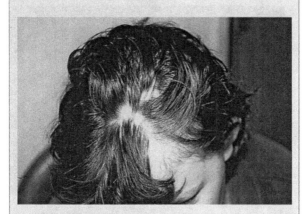

Fig. 2.17 This patient has both a postpartum telogen effluvium and recurrent alopecia areata.

Continued on p. 28

2 A middle-aged woman reported significant diffuse hair loss over a 6–8-week period (Fig. 2.18). An inadequate history led to the loss being attributed to the use of a particular shampoo.

Further expert opinion revealed that the patient had lost over 16 kg in weight after using dexphenfluramine for a

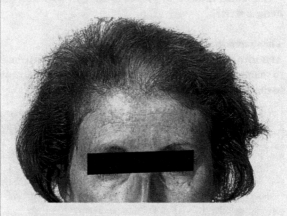

Fig. 2.18 Diffuse loss affecting primarily the temporal/vertical areas may be difficult to diagnose; it is never due to the use of cosmetic products.

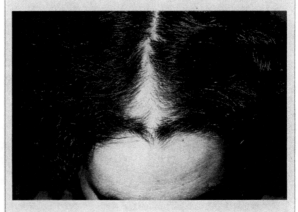

Fig. 2.19 Early androgenetic alopecia in a 30-year-old woman; this can be misdiagnosed since neither party wishes to contemplate 'baldness'.

Continued on p. 29

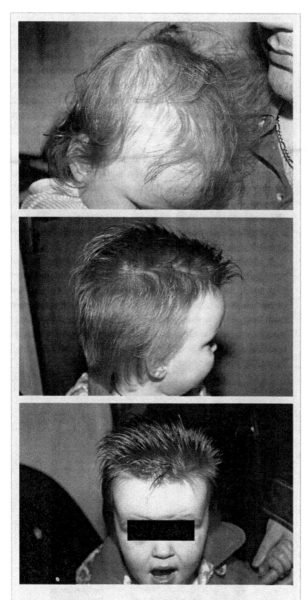

Fig. 2.20 Hair loss due to telogen effluvium and subsequent regrowth following surgery and postoperative infection.

Continued on p. 30

crash diet, prescribed by her doctor. Hair pull revealed the presence of a raised number of telogen hairs. Reassurance and adequate diet led to complete recovery.

3 A 30-year-old woman reported diffuse hair loss over many months, again attributed to the use of a topical hair care product (Fig. 2.19). Local opinion agreed. Two further expert opinions concurred that the patient had early onset of androgenetic alopecia of which there was a strong family history.

4 A 3-year-old child suffered diffuse hair loss. Informed and experienced primary care opinion attributed this to recent surgery and a postoperative infection. Hair regrowth was obvious within 3 months, but the new hair had different characteristics—it was thicker and straighter. This is a recognized phenomenon and is probably partially due to synchronous growth (Fig. 2.20).

5 A mother reported a localized area of baldness in her young child, which she attributed to the use of a shampoo (Fig. 2.21). Initial assessment suggested alopecia areata, but expert examination revealed a localized area on the vertex with hairs of different lengths visible and under a hand lens suggestions of fractures could be seen. A diagnosis of self-mutilation (trichotillomania) was established and later confirmed by observation.

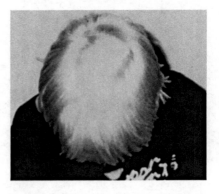

Fig. 2.21 An area of hair loss which mimics alopecia areata but which in fact is traumatic (trichotillomania).

Scalp examination

The scalp must be examined all over to determine hair density, distribution, quality and pattern of loss (Fig. 2.22). It is essential to determine if the hair loss is:

1 diffuse or focal; and

2 scarring or non-scarring.

The pattern of loss may be diagnostic, but the physician should be cautions that apparent loss may in fact be an extreme of normality. Figure 2.23 illustrates a normal high

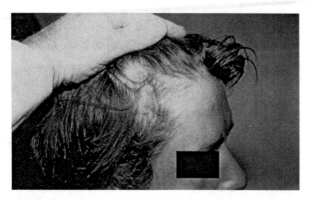

Fig. 2.22 The hair must be examined all over the scalp to assess the hair density; this woman has a reduced density in the temporal regions.

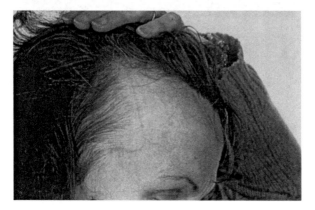

Fig. 2.23 This patient has a normal high forehead which mimics androgenetic alopecia.

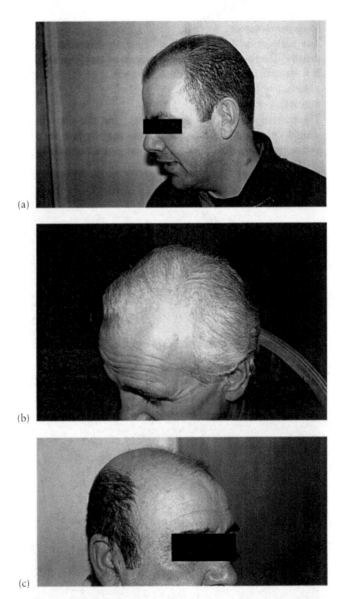

(a)

(b)

(c)

Fig. 2.24 Different patterns of hair loss in male androgenetic alopecia: (a) bitemporal recession in a man of 23, (b) extensive loss with sparing of the occiput, (c) severe bitemporal recession and diffuse loss.

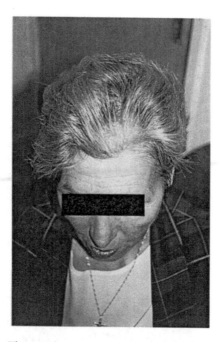

Fig. 2.25 The typical appearance of androgenetic alopecia in a female, with preservation of the frontal margin and reduced density.

forehead mimicking androgenetic alopecia. Androgenetic alopecia in males affects the vertex but not the occiput (Fig. 2.24). In females, the loss is more diffuse and on the top of the scalp but with preservation of the hair line even in severe cases (Fig. 2.25).

Parting the hair (Fig. 2.26) reveals the overall density.

Diffuse hair loss on the back and sides of the head suggests a systemic cause (Fig. 2.27). Diffuse alopecia with some bitemporal recession is likely to be a telogen effluvium).

Patchy alopecia may be caused by AA, tinea capitis, trichotillomania (self-mutilation) or a cicatrizing (scarring) alopecia.

Focal hair loss may be either unifocal (Fig. 2.28) or multifocal (Fig. 2.29).

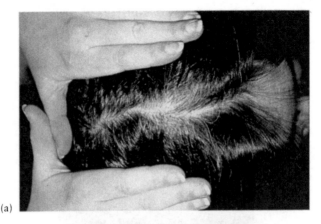

(a)

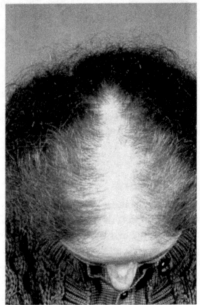

(b)

Fig. 2.26 Parting the hair reveals the overall density.

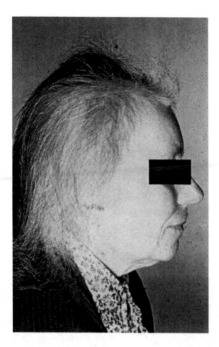

Fig. 2.27 Severe diffuse loss. In this case the patient has a telogen effluvium due to iron deficiency anaemia.

Traction alopecias are characterized by loss at the margins of the hair (Fig. 2.30).

Some useful reference guides are available to assess androgenetic alopecia (see Figs 2.44 & 2.45).

The scalp should be examined to determine whether underlying scalp pathology is implicated as a cause. Possibilities include infestations (erythema and scaling), infections (Fig. 2.31), scarring (cicatrizing) alopecias, atrophy and obvious neoplasia (Fig. 2.32), (benign and malignant).

Specific examination

THE HAIR PULL TEST
This, after detailed inspection of the scalp, is the most important part of the scalp examination.

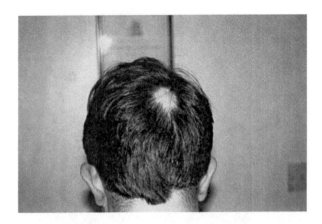

Fig. 2.28 Aplasia cutis.

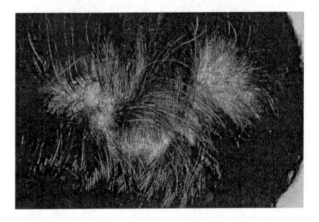

Fig. 2.29 Multifocal loss in Darrier's disease.

With the thumb and forefinger gently pull on the hair (Fig. 2.33). This is repeated in various sections over the whole of the scalp, six to eight times in total.

If the proximal ends of the hairs obtained on a hair pull are examined by the naked eye or hand lens in a good light against a dark background, one of three findings will be evident:

• normal telogen bulbs;

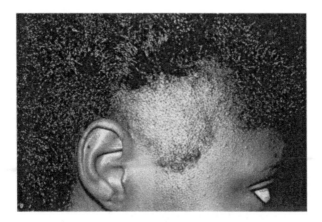

Fig. 2.30 Traction alopecias are characterized by hair loss at the margins: hairs of different lengths are almost conclusively diagnostic.

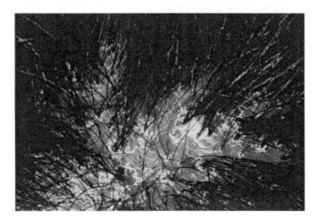

Fig. 2.31 Erythema and discharge accompanying tufted folliculitis.

- broken hairs;
- abnormal anagen hairs.

In the vast majority of cases, only normal telogen bulbs are seen. This is to be expected on examination of a normal scalp. The telogen hair is easy to recognize. To the naked eye, it appears to have a dry, hard, club-shaped bulb (Fig. 2.34). If in doubt as to the nature of these hairs, examina-

37

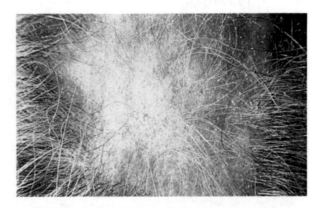

Fig. 2.32 Hair loss due to neoplastic deposit.

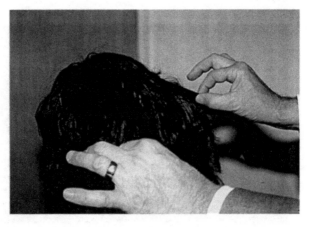

Fig. 2.33 The hair pull test should exert only moderate traction.

tion under a hand lens is useful (Fig. 2.35). There is no ter-minal hair shaft pigment.

Normally, a total of 2–5 telogen hairs will be obtained in a hair pull test, depending on when the hair was last sham-pooed and styled: the more time which has passed since the last shampooing, the more telogen hairs will be obtained in a hair pull.

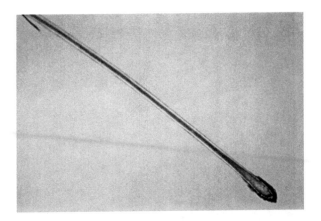

Fig. 2.34 A typical telogen hair terminates in a club-shaped root.

Any broken hairs may be the 'exclamation point' hairs associated with alopecia areata (Fig. 2.36). These can be found along the margins of the patches.

If the hair is fragile through either cosmetic damage or a hair shaft abnormality, gentle pulling near the base of the hairs may leave fragments on the fingers.

An active telogen effluvium is generally easy to recognize since, in this situation, the number of hairs in a hair pull will be at least three or four times normal. In very severe cases many obviously telogen hairs will be easily pulled.

If light microscopic examination (see below) of the proximal ends of the hairs obtained on a hair pull reveals long succulent bulbs, these are probably anagen hairs (Fig. 2.37), and the loss is due to an anagen effluvium or loose anagen syndrome. Normal anagen hairs cannot be dislodged by the degree of traction generated by a simple hair pull, but require forcible plucking. Pulling on anagen hair is painful and will generally cause breakage before the hair shaft can be extracted.

Any number of anagen hairs present on a hair pull is abnormal.

LIGHT MICROSCOPY

For those interested, simple light microscopic analysis of the

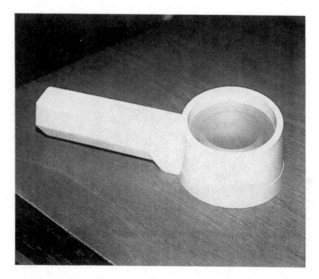

Fig. 2.35 A hand lens is a useful diagnostic tool.

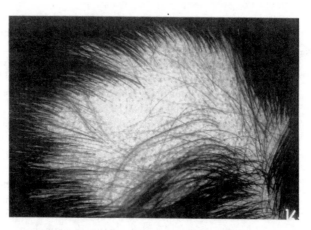

Fig. 2.36 'Exclamation point' hairs, i.e. broken hairs usually found at the margins of the lesions, are typical of alopecia areata.

hair shaft is most useful in assessing hair shaft damage and congenital or acquired abnormalities of the shaft (Fig. 2.38).

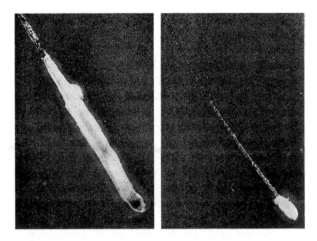

Fig. 2.37 Hairs extracted by a hair pluck: anagen hairs (left), telogen hairs (right). The anagen hair is sticky and will adhere to the underside of a glass slide.

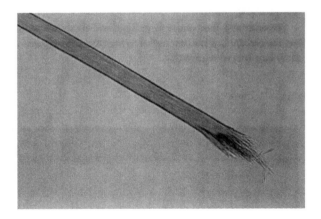

Fig. 2.38 Split end seen under the light microscope.

Hairs can be mounted on sticky tape, or between two slides taped together.

Light microscopy is also useful in assessing the relative diameters of hairs. In a normal scalp, terminal hairs are of variable diameter, but in women with androgenetic alopecia this variability is exaggerated in involved areas, and a mosaic of miniaturized and normal-sized terminal hair shafts can be seen.

Quantitative analysis of hair loss

Determining the actual number of hairs shed per day (Fig. 2.39) can be helpful to corroborate the loss, or to reassure the patient that the process is either stable or resolving. Since shampooing and grooming practices vary from day to day and each affects hair shedding, averaging the daily hair shedding over at least a week's span is important. Patients are asked to collect all hairs shed in the shower or sink, or on brush, comb, pillow and so on, daily for 7 days in individual plastic bags, and then to count and average these. Normally, the daily loss is 50–80 hairs per day: the 100 hairs per day quoted widely in the literature appears in practice to be in excess of that lost by the average young, healthy person. In an active telogen effluvium, however, several hundred hairs may be shed each day, which is to be expected if the telogen percentage increases from a normal of 10% to 30–40% (Fig. 2.40).

Performing a hair count is tedious and time-consuming for the patient but is often useful to monitor the progress of their hair loss or regrowth.

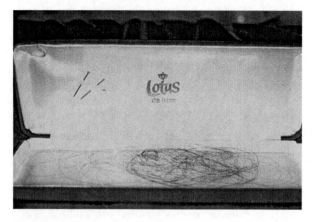

Fig. 2.39 One day's normal hair loss.

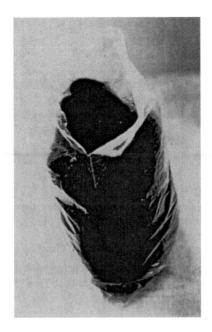

Fig. 2.40 One year's normal hair loss.

HAIR GROWTH WINDOW

One interesting method of assessing the rate of growth is to monitor growth on a small shaved area of the scalp occluded for up to 2 weeks. The patch is removed and the length of the hairs measured. Normal weekly growth is about 2.5 mm. This is a useful 'public relations' measure for demonstrating to patients that their hair is indeed growing. Photography is similarly reassuring but is not necessarily an accurate tool under the conditions that apply in office practice.

THE HAIR PLUCK

This is not an examination relevant to most conditions seen in everyday practice, but it should be performed in cases where one wishes to establish an anagen/telogen ratio or to evaluate whether any catagen hairs are present. It consists of grasping 40–50 hairs by forceps and extracting them — a painful procedure. It may be very damaging to the hair shaft, and the procedure may reveal apparently dystrophic roots.

SCALP BIOPSIES

These are only of relevance when a scarring alopecia is a possibility or where there is serious doubt about the diagnosis — in a suspected self-mutilation (trichotillomania), for example. Follicular structures can be identified and reliable information on the anagen:telogen ratio determined. Inflammatory changes and fibrosis can be detected.

Laboratory investigations

The following simple investigations may be useful in the assessment of the causes of alopecia:

FULL BLOOD COUNT/ESR

Severe or persistent anaemia is a recognized cause of telogen effluvium. A raised ESR may indicate relevant systemic disease.

FERRITIN/SERUM IRON DETERMINATION/
ZINC LEVELS

There is significant controversy whether low ferritin levels in the absence of anaemia is a genuine cause of hair loss.

Congenital zinc deficiency is, however, recognized as a cause of poor hair growth in children, with abnormal forms of hair and premature breakage. The effects in adults of low zinc concentrations are more difficult to establish.

THYROID FUNCTION TESTS

Hypothyroidism is accepted as a factor in telogen effluvium (Fig. 2.41), since the biological hair factory is susceptible to metabolic disturbance. Correction of thyroid levels usually sees a gradual regrowth.

RENAL AND HEPATIC FUNCTION TESTS

These should be performed where there is a suggestion of a systemic disease. Chronic disorders can cause a general reduction in hair follicle metabolism, leading to a diffuse alopecia.

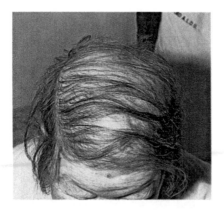

Fig. 2.41 Hair loss in severe hypothyroidism.

VDLR

Syphilis in some parts of the world still constitutes a recognized cause of hair loss.

SERUM ANDROGENS

Androgen levels, including total testosterone, should be monitored where disorders of androgenic function are suspected; however, the results are of no routine value in assessing androgenetic alopecia.

Gross disturbance of androgen function affects hair follicles susceptible to dihydrotestosterone and produces a male pattern androgenetic alopecia. In women, the relatively low oestrogen production in later life allows the effects of inherent androgens to appear, including hair thinning; HRT does not appear to reverse the effects, however.

Androgenetic alopecia

Throughout the world this is the most frequent cause of hair loss, affecting both men and women. It is genetically determined, being an autosomal dominant with variable penetrance (Figs 2.42–48). It generally presents from the second decade onward in men and the third decade in women.

Under the influence of androgens the follicles in the temporal, frontal and vertex areas progressively show a short-

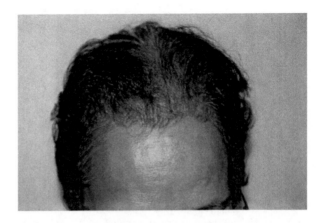

Fig. 2.42 Androgenetic alopecia: characteristic female pattern with preservation of hair line.

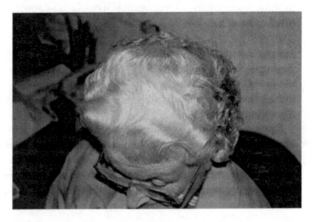

Fig. 2.43 Androgenetic alopecia: characteristic female pattern. At this age the density is almost expected.

ening of the anagen phase, accompanied by miniaturization of the hair follicles. A greater percentage of hairs will be persistently in telogen, leading to accumulating loss. The pattern of this loss has been defined by Ludwig in women and Hamilton in men (Figs 2.44 & 2.45).

The hair cycle of the scalp is affected by androgenetic alopecia in both sexes. The percentage of hairs in anagen

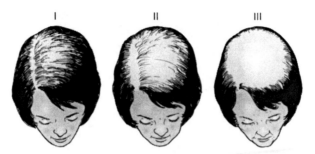

Fig. 2.44 The Ludwig pattern and the Hamilton pattern (see below) are typical of hair loss in the sexes; there is considerable variation, however, as the hairs minaturize.

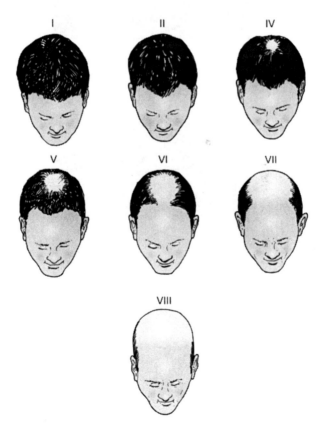

Fig. 2.45 The Hamilton classification of scalp hair distribution.

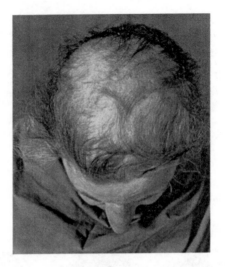

Fig. 2.46 Androgenetic alopecia: characteristic female pattern with obvious preservation of hair line—Ludwig III.

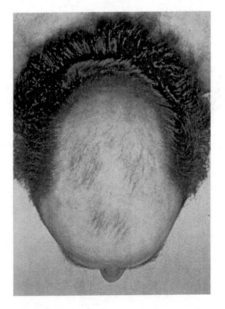

Fig. 2.47 Androgenetic alopecia: characteristic male pattern— Hamilton grade VIII.

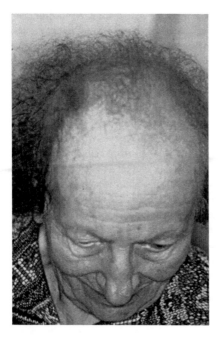

Fig. 2.48 Androgenetic alopecia: severe type in a woman of 80 years of age. In extreme old age this may be synonymous with 'involutional' alopecia.

and the duration of anagen both diminish in areas affected by androgenetic alopecia, resulting in shorter hairs. More hairs are in telogen, and remain in telogen for longer periods; telogen hairs are much more subject to loss with daily trauma than anagen hairs are, and this affects the apparent density of the hair.

Male androgenetic alopecia

In men who develop androgenetic alopecia the hair loss may begin any time after puberty, when serum androgen levels rise above the low level found in normal young boys.

The first change is usually a bitemporal recession, which is seen in 96% of sexually mature Caucasian males, including those men not destined to progress to further hair loss. The density of hair in a given pattern of loss tends to diminish with age. There is no way of predicting the pattern of hair loss in a young man with early androgenetic alopecia. In general, those who begin losing hair in the second decade are those in whom the alopecia will progress the most extensively. In some men, initial male-pattern hair loss may be delayed until the late third to the fourth decade. All the hairs in an affected area may eventually (though not necessarily) become involved in the miniaturization process and may with time cover the region with fine vellus hair. Pigment production ceases with progressive miniaturization. The scalp may appear bald long before vellus hair is lost.

There are racial as well as age-related differences in the incidence or pattern of hair loss in male androgenetic alopecia. Oriental and Native American men are more likely than Caucasians to preserve the frontal hairline and have less extensive baldness. African-American men may also have a lower incidence and extent of baldness, with decreased frequency of frontoparietal loss.

Virility is not a marker for male-pattern baldness: only 2% of androgens are available for deposition in tissues such as the hair follicles, the remaining 98% being protein-bound.

Female androgenetic alopecia

Hair loss in women affected by androgenetic alopecia is likely to be first noticed in the late twenties through the early forties, compared with the late teens and twenties in men. It is particularly likely at times of hormonal change, i.e. institution or discontinuation of oral contraceptive pills, the postpartum period and the perimenopausal and early postmenopausal periods. In most women with androgenetic alopecia there is no evidence of abnormal androgen production. Bitemporal recession occurs at sexual maturation in ~90% of females as well as in most men, but is generally much less noticeable in women.

Women rarely go completely bald. The end result of the condition in women is a visible decrease in density of hair, rather than baldness, in the affected areas.

Most women in middle to old age who present with hair thinning have androgenetic alopecia, often made worse by other factors, such as iron deficiency or low thyroid activity.

- At age 25, 25% of all men will have some obvious hair loss.
- At age 50, 50% of all men will have some obvious hair loss.
- Hair loss starts, on average, 10 years later in women than men.

Management of androgenetic alopecia

Many, if not most men accept that they may go bald. Many others desperately seek a cure! Unfortunately there is no cure for androgenetic alopecia at present. The treatment of the condition is fraught with myths. Stress, diet and topical hair care products have all been blamed: all are blameless.

It is essential to remember that a small but important minority have dysmorphophobia regarding their appearance and may be depressed enough by their hair loss to attempt suicide. Guiding patients with severe androgenetic alopecia to specialist help is part of the primary care role.

Surgical treatments are beyond the scope of this book, but the recently introduced mini- and micro-grafts have been increasingly successful, giving a natural re-growth pattern. Previous punch biopsy methods were cosmetically less satisfactory and some unsuccessful attempts resulted in failure and residual hyperpigmentation (Fig. 2.49).

Wigs, which can be woven with pre-existing hair, are sometimes satisfactory. Patients should however be counselled that suturing of wigs may result in traction alopecia.

Antiandrogen treatments, although logically the treatment of choice, are precluded in men because of their side-effects. Cyproterone acetate in combination with ethinyl oestradiol may bring about hair regrowth in women. Drugs with antiandrogenic activity showing promise include Finesteride (previously marketed as Proscar for benign prostatic hypertrophy), which is taken orally at a 1 mg daily dose. It is a 5-alpha reductase inhibitor and reduces the levels of dihydrotestosterone in the scalp. It has just received FDA approval for use in men.

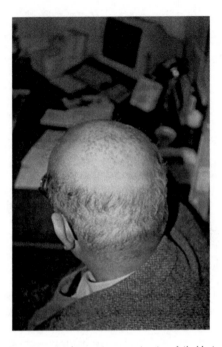

Fig. 2.49 Postoperative hyperpigmentation in a failed hair transplantation.

Many other systemic preparations, such as cyclosporin, may lead to hypertrichosis. These are clearly not acceptable as routine therapy for hair regrowth.

No government currently supports reimbursable treatment for androgenetic alopecia. A 2% topical preparation of minoxidil is currently available in many countries, either on prescription or over the counter; if treatment is commenced early enough it may lead to up to 30% conversion of vellus hairs to terminal hairs. Only some 10% of men will experience full regrowth, however. Recently a 5% solution of this drug has gained FDA approval. According to various sources, at best it may stop the loss in about 80% of users, whilst 30% will see some downy growth after three or four months and 30% some visible growth. Minoxidil treatment has to be used continuously—for life!

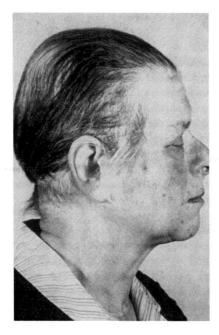

Fig. 2.50 Diffuse alopecia of uncertain cause in a woman aged 74 years.

Diffuse alopecia

Diffuse hair loss is, after androgenetic alopecia, the commonest type of hair loss. The whole scalp is affected, although a great deal of hair has to be shed before the condition becomes visible (Fig. 2.50).

Diffuse loss of hair is seldom acute in the true sense of the word. The rapidity of visibility depends more on the actual numbers of hairs entering telogen and being shed.

Telogen effluvium

Diffuse alopecia with excessive telogen hair shedding from normal follicles has been associated with a variety of hormonal and nutritional factors, drugs, chemicals, systemic and local cutaneous disease, and (possibly) psychological stress; it is also frequently seen in young children. Some of these associations, such as a postpartum effluvium, are well documented; others, though often quoted, are less well established. The condition is less common in males than in females.

Postpartum hair loss

Postpartum alopecia is probably the most widely recognized form of excessive telogen hair shedding and most new mothers are not totally surprised when it occurs. It is generally thought that the high oestrogen levels of pregnancy are responsible for prolongation of the anagen phase, and a synchrony of hair growth. The mass reversal to telogen as oestrogen declines is thought to be responsible for this effect. Rarely it may continue into a chronic telogen effluvium.

Hormonal factors

Alterations in hormone levels, especially those of the thyroid and sex hormones, influence the hair follicle. The associated alopecia usually disappears when hormonal homeostasis is re-established (unless androgenetic alopecia is also present).

Diffuse hair loss may be present as the only symptom of **hypothyroidism**. Deficiency of thyroid hormone is probably responsible for the alopecia, which is characterized by a decrease in the anagen:telogen ratio. There is no known correlation between thyroid hormone levels and degree of alopecia.

Oral contraceptives

Hair loss whilst using oral contraceptives has been reported; so too has diffuse alopecia on cessation of oral contraceptives. A history of previous postpartum hair loss is variably present. Studies of the effects of oral contraceptives on the hair cycle have proved inconclusive.

Nutritional factors

WEIGHT LOSS

Crash dieting or chronic nutritional deprivation (starvation or alcoholism) may result in diffuse hair shedding, usually because an increased number of hairs are entering telogen. Hair loss may recur with subsequent diets.

Prognosis for regrowth after discontinuation of the diet is

generally good. Significant reductions in T3 have been noted in dieting patients, and it is possible that diet-related reduction of thyroid activity may contribute to hair loss.

Advanced protein deficiency results in fine, brittle and sparse hair. An increase of telogen hairs was found in elderly individuals who were protein-deficient, as well as in children with classic protein-calorie malnutrition.

IRON DEFICIENCY

The role of iron deficiency in telogen effluvium is controversial. Iron deficiency, with or without anaemia, has been reported to be present in as many as 72% of women with diffuse alopecia associated with an increased percentage of telogen hairs. It is thought that iron deficiency results in decreased depot iron and tissue iron well before anaemia is manifest. Other reports indicate that there is no correlation between low ferritin levels and established alopecia. In general practice the number of women with very low ferritin levels is not matched by complaints of hair loss.

ZINC DEFICIENCY

It is recognized that symptoms of zinc deficiency include hair loss.

Zinc deficiency may be either hereditary or acquired. In the former case there is an inborn defect of zinc absorption (Fig. 2.51). Acquired deficiency may result from a lack of dietary zinc or long-continued parenteral alimentation.

Fever

Postfebrile alopecia has been described as an increased telogen hair shedding beginning anywhere from 2 to 5 months after a febrile illness.

The cause is probably a response of the hair bulb to systemic or local mediators resulting in premature shutdown of a proportion of follicles and a consequent increase in the numbers entering telogen.

Systemic illness

Various systemic illnesses, including Crohn's disease and hepatic disease, have been reported to be associated with diffuse hair loss (Fig. 2.52). Some, such as syphilis, may be characterized by diffuse telogen hair shedding as the

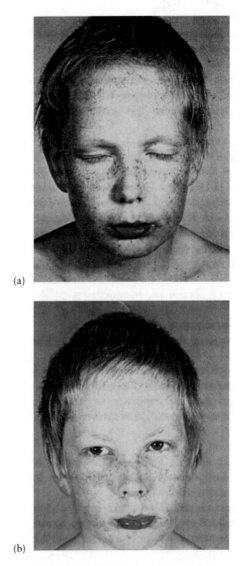

(a)

(b)

Fig. 2.51 Congenital zinc deficiency (a) before treatment, note the closed eyes (photophobia), and (b) after treatment.

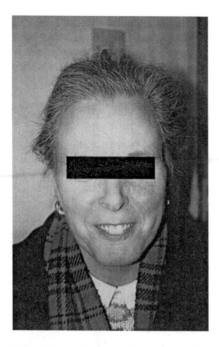

Fig. 2.52 This lady has hair loss after chemotherapy. In her case it was due to a telogen rather than anagen effluvium.

presenting symptom, and lymphoproliferative disorders have also been associated with telogen hair shedding. Inflammatory bowel disease has been associated with chronic hair loss.

Surgery

Diffuse hair loss (telogen effluvium) after surgery has been described. The cause of hair loss in these instances is not known. A specific postoperative localized pressure alopecia may occur, probably caused by pressure-induced ischaemia.

Stress and alopecia

Psychological stress is widely held to be a common cause of hair loss. It must be remembered that hair loss itself is very stressful to most of the individuals who experience it, and that it can often be difficult if not impossible to determine which came first, stress or hair loss. In all probability, though in the absence of hard data, it may be said that psychogenic alopecia does occur but only in a few of those complaining of hair loss. Alopecia areata is often implicated in this type of scenario.

CASE STUDY

This patient (Fig. 2.53) reported severe hair loss at age 56, some 8 months after being made redundant and suffering severe depression. He went on to develop alopecia universalis (loss of all body hair). He had no past history of the disease. The temporal association seems overwhelming.

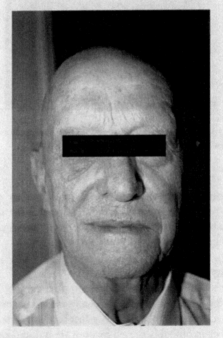

Fig. 2.53 Alopecia universalis developing after severe depressive illness. The social effects are sometimes devastating.

Drugs and alopecia

A large number of drugs have been reported to cause, or possibly cause, diffuse alopecia (Table 2.1).

Table 2.1 Drugs and chemicals reported to cause or possibly cause telogen hair loss.

Allopurinol
Androgens (danazol)
Angiotensin-converting enzyme inhibitors (captopril, enalapril)
Anticholesterolaemic drugs (clofibrate, triparanol)
Anticoagulants (coumarin, dextran, heparin, heparinoids)
Antimitotic agents (colchicine, methotrexate)
Antithyroid medications (carbimaxole, methylthiouracil, propylthiouracil)
Benzimidazoles (albendazole, mebendazole)
Beta blockers (systemic: metoprolol, propranolol; topical ophthalmic: betaxalol, levobunolol, timolol)
Bromocriptine
Cimetidine
Gold
Immunoglobulin
Interferon (alpha, gamma)
Levodopa
Methysergide
Minoxidil
Oral contraceptives
Proguanil
Psychotropic medications (amphetamines, desipramine, dixyrazine, fluoxetine, imipramine, lithium, tranylcypromine, valproic acid)
Pyridostigmine bromide
Retinoids
Sulfasalazine
Terfenadine
Vitamin A

Prognosis for hair regrowth after the drug is stopped is generally good.

Amphetamines used for weight loss have been incriminated as a cause of a type of hair loss temporally consistent with telogen effluvium.

Involutional alopecia

Involutional (senescent, senile) alopecia is found in both sexes and is defined as diffuse hair thinning occurring after the age of 50 years with a negative family history of male-pattern baldness. The pattern often closely resembles that of androgenetic alopecia.

Prognosis for hair regrowth is generally good provided that the cause of the telogen hair shedding can be found and eliminated, and that the patient does not have associated androgenetic alopecia.

Anagen effluvium
A premature interruption of growth in anagen causes an increased proportion of hairs to enter telogen. When anagen restarts between 2 and 4 months later the telogen hairs are literally pushed out of their follicles.

By far the commonest cause of the condition in practice is chemotherapy.

Alopecia areata
A sudden patchy loss of hairs may be due to the condition known as **alopecia areata**, which is relatively common: as many as one person in a thousand may expect to suffer from it at some time. The cause is unknown and occasionally it becomes very widespread and severe. It is considered by some to have an autoimmune mechanism but there may be an external trigger. The role of stress is debatable. There is a variably reported association with thyroid disease. Related autoimmune disorders include Hashimoto's disease, pernicious anaemia and rheumatoid arthritis. It is relatively common in children (Fig. 2.54).

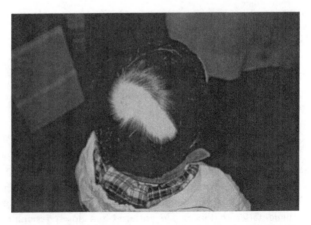

Fig. 2.54 A case of alopecia areata in a child. Full recovery ensued.

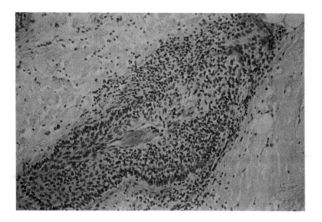

Fig. 2.55 A catagen hair follicle surrounded by a lymphocyte swarm. Courtesy of Dr A. McDonagh, Sheffield, UK.

It is characterized by a persistent lymphocyte infiltrate in and around the hair follicles (Fig. 2.55), sometimes associated with Langerhans cells.

The condition is easily identified by microscopic examination of the shed hairs, which characteristically look like exclamation marks. A hand lens is probably adequate but a simple microscope is obviously far better.

Occasionally in practice, a severe acute alopecia areata may be encountered. In such a case, touching the side of the patient's head may lead to a sudden loss of vast handfuls of hair, revealing almost bald scalp beneath. This comes as a shock to patient and physician alike, and must be met with a full explanation.

Nail changes are common in alopecia areata patients, varying from marked alteration of the nails to fine pitting.

Management of alopecia areata

In most cases, particularly where it is localized, the condition should be managed conservatively. Reassurance should be given, together with periodic re-examination and photographing to show progress. Usually the hair reappears without treatment, although in persistent cases in adults intralesional steroid injections (triamcinolone) may help.

Sometimes the condition becomes severe and/or recurrent, and the patient may ultimate even lose eyebrows and lashes (**alopecia totalis**) or all body hair (**alopecia universalis**) (Fig. 2.56). In such cases the prognosis is pessimistic. Events may resolve slowly but an exacerbation is inevitably dramatic.

Overall, about 50% of patients developing alopecia areata before puberty will probably eventually become bald (see R. Dawber & A. Van Neste 1995, *Hair & Scalp Disorders:* Dunitz.)

There is no really effective drug treatment for severe alopecia areata. A diverse approach has included the use of irritants such as dithranol and of systemic steroids and PUVA. Treatment with immune enhancers (i.e. substances inducing contact allergic dermatitis, such as diphencyprone) is occasionally useful but has an unpleasant side-effect profile.

Topical minoxidil with or without oral steroids for short periods has been used. Cyclosporin may have dramatic effects but they are usually temporary.

In deciding how to treat alopecia areata, the age of onset and severity are key factors. Prepubertal onset of severe nature should warrant referral to a specialist centre, but

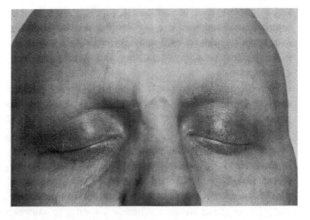

Fig. 2.56 Alopecia universalis.

with appropriate counselling regarding prognosis and help in social adjustment.

Alopecia areata and white hair
The myth of 'going grey overnight' almost certainly arises from a variant of alopecia areata. In the case illustrated in Fig. 2.57, the hairs were originally a mixture of black and white. The pigmented hairs were suddenly lost over a few days or weeks but the unpigmented, medullated hairs were, curiously, spared. With regrowth the previous 'pepper-and-salt' mixture was restored.

Patchy loss of facial hair, including eyebrows, eye lashes and beard, may be the sole sign of alopecia areata, or associated with obvious scalp loss (Fig. 2.58).

Alopecia due to cosmetic problems
Apparent hair loss caused by cosmetic problems is invariably the result of hair breakage. This may be due to the rapid induction of severe weathering and cortical disruption from over-processing with chemical agents such as permanent wave solutions or bleaches. Alternatively it may be caused by physical abuse such as traction, or overheating with hair dryers. There are certain abnormalities of the hair shaft that may contribute to this hair breakage (Fig. 2.59).

Alopecia due to hair shaft disorders
Abnormalities of the hair shaft can be either inherited or acquired, and may be caused by underlying disease. Congenital abnormalities of the hair shaft are very rare, affecting only about 1 in 10000 of the population. The practising physician will, however, see more hair abnormalities associated with cosmetic problems than almost all other disorders combined. The interested observer of the human head may be surprised at the level of damage that can be wrought (Fig. 2.60).

Abnormal hair shaft structure, whatever the cause, can lead to apparent hair loss (Fig. 2.61) since such shafts are liable to be brittle and break off. Examination of the hair shaft by light microscopy can be useful in establishing a diagnosis.

It has to be remembered that in any head of normal hair

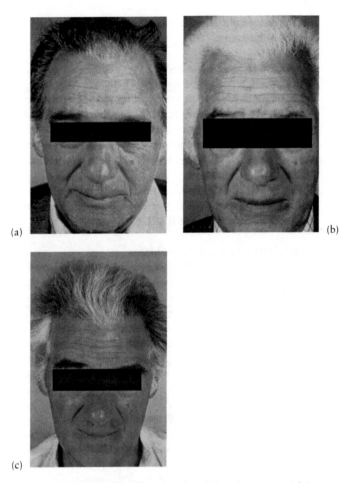

(a)

(b)

(c)

Fig. 2.57 Abrupt loss of pigmented hair led to almost 'overnight' greying, but the hair colour spontaneously reverted to normal as new hair grew during the following few weeks. Courtesy of Dr D. Fenton, London, UK.

there will be some abnormal hairs with twists and irregularities. It is often reported on the basis of a few isolated microscopic examinations that a patient has a congenital abnormality of the hair shaft. Only when hairs from all over the scalp are consistently reported as abnormal, however, should this diagnosis be entertained.

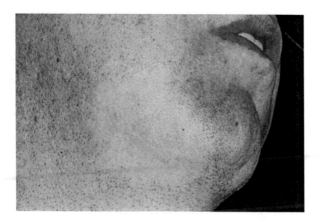

Fig. 2.58 Patchy loss of facial hair may occur in AA.

There are four main types of hair shaft abnormality:
- fractures;
- irregularities;
- coiling and twisting; and
- extraneous matter.

In everyday practice, the commonest abnormality of the hair shaft is acquired from inappropriate cosmetic treatments. Perming, bleaching or a combination of these, allied to excessive use of the hair dryer, can lead to a mass of friable hair which can break under further 'stress'.

People with African (Negroid) hair have exceptional susceptibility to hair-shaft damage from chemical and physical trauma. Relaxing (straightening) is very common and places even further stress on the shaft. A tendency to knotting may further add to the fragility of friable hair.

The following show some of the rare hair shaft abnormalities that may be associated with hair breakage and apparent hair loss.

Classification of hair shaft defects

FRACTURES OF THE HAIR SHAFT

Transverse
Trichorrhexis nodosa (Fig. 2.62), congenital and acquired

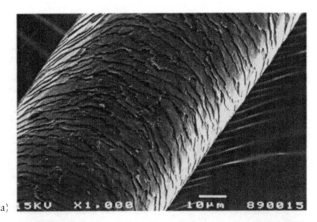

(a)

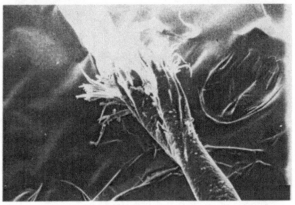

(b)

Fig. 2.59 (a) Hair shaft showing minimal weathering of the cuticle. (b) Severe weathering in a hair with the congenital abnormality pili torti.

Trichoclasis
Trichoschisis, including trichothiodystrophy
Trichorrhexis invaginata, including bamboo hair

Oblique fracture

Tapered fracture
Longitudinal
Trichoptilosis.

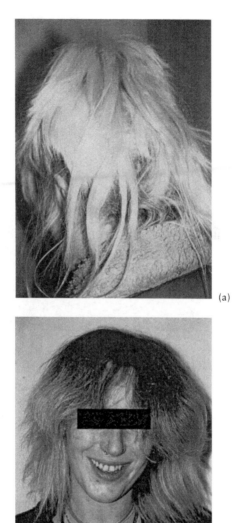

(a)

(b)

Fig. 2.60 Gross weathering due to repeated bleaching allied to poor hair care in general.

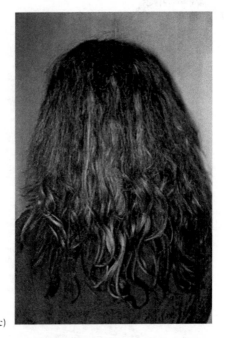

(c)

Fig. 2.60 *Continued* (c) Repeated bleaching with 60% peroxide resulting in gross weathering over many years.

HAIR SHAFT COILING AND TWISTING

Pili torti, including corkscrew hair and Menkes' syndrome
Woolly hair, including acquired progressive kinking, therapy-induced kinking, and whisker hair
Trichonodosis (knotted hair)
Circle hairs

IRREGULARITIES OF THE HAIR SHAFT

• Longitudinal ridging and grooving, including loose anagen syndrome and congenital hypotrichosis
• Uncombable hair or pili trianguli et canaliculi or spun glass hair, including straight hair naevus
• Pili multigemini and pili bifurcati
• Trichostasis spinulosa
• Pili annulati
• Pseudo pili annulati
• Pilar melanin clumps, in Chédiak–Higashi syndrome

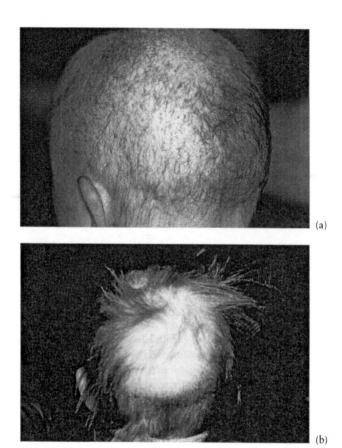

(a)

(b)

Fig. 2.61 Monilethrix is a congenital abnormality which can result in apparent hair loss due to breakage. (b) Hair loss due to breakage associated with pili torti, a congenital abnormality of the hair shaft accompanied by twisting.

- Monilethrix
- Pseudo monilethrix, tapered hairs, including Pohl-Pinkus mark, bayonet hairs, tapered newly growing anagen hairs, and trichomalacia
- Bubble hairs
- Intermittent hair-follicle dystrophy
- Acquired eyelash trichomegaly

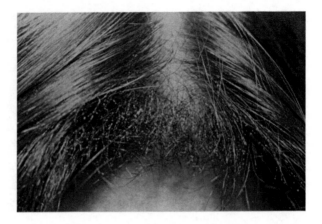

Fig. 2.62 Clinical appearance of trichorrhexis nodosa.

Weathering

The term 'weathering' is applied to the mechanical and chemical breakdown of the free end of the hair shaft that occurs with time. Long scalp hairs that have been growing for several years are particularly subject to weathering.

The hair shaft is reasonably resistant to 'normal' wear and tear. Repeated mechanical stress (wet combing, heat) and chemical damage (perms, bleaching) can, however, result in premature disruption of the cuticle and cortex. The effects of these procedures include accelerated loss of cuticle scales, and ultimately exposure and subsequent fraying of the cortical fibres.

Figures 2.63–65 illustrate varying degrees of excessive cosmetic weathering. Ultimately breakage can occur, with inevitable apparent hair loss.

SPECIFIC FORMS OF WEATHERING

Fractures of the hair shaft

Certain specific types of weathering are associated with fractures of the hair shaft (Fig. 2.66).

Fractures of the hair shaft can result in apparent loss. A detailed history including use of chemical and physical processes on the hair is essential to assess the degree of accelerated weathering that may have occurred. Careful

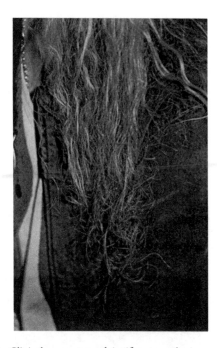

Fig. 2.63 Clinical appearance of significant weathering.

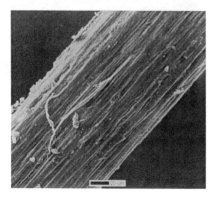

Fig. 2.64 Moderate damage to the hair shaft due to weathering.

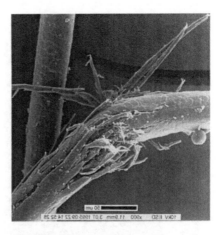

Fig. 2.65 Severe damage due to weathering.

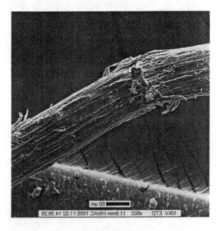

Fig. 2.66 Trichoclasis is a specific fracture of the hair shaft associated with cosmetic weathering.

clinical examination is required, including the assessment of serial samples of hair from different regions of the scalp. Feeling the hair texture is important, as irregularities of the shaft can often be detected by tactile information.

The following are recognized as clinical entities, but each represents only a specific morphological form of weathering.

Trichorrhexis nodosa

Trichorrhexis nodosa (see Fig. 2.62) is the most common expanded fracture of the hair shaft (Fig. 2.67). It appears along the hair shaft as a patchy loss of cuticle cells and is invariably the result of weathering due to cosmetic processes. The expanded areas are composed of splayed-out cortical fibres, which resemble the frayed ends of a rope.

The basic cause of trichorrhexis nodosa is mechanical or chemical trauma but inherent weakness of the hair shaft, such as sulphur deficiency (trichothiodystrophy, Fig. 2.68), may contribute.

Excessive physical insults such as over-energetic brushing, backcombing, stressed hairstyles, tight braids, ponytails, hair weaving, the application of heat (Fig. 2.69) and prolonged exposure to ultraviolet light can be contributory factors.

Clinical examination shows nodes seen as grey-white or yellow specks on the affected hair shafts. Hairs tend to frac-

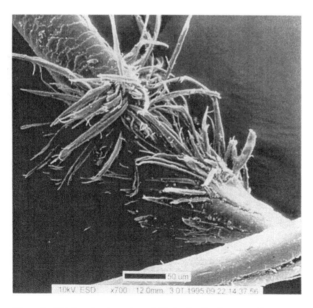

Fig. 2.67 Trichorrhexis nodosa. This is classically caused by excessive heat resulting in rupture of the cortex.

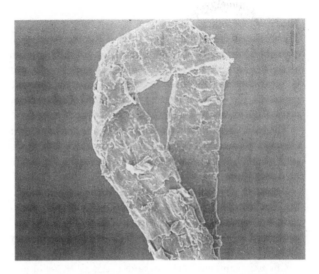

Fig. 2.68 The flattened, tape-like appearance of the hair shaft in trichothiodystrophy.

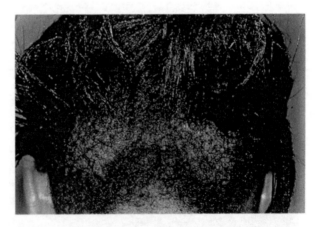

Fig. 2.69 Hair breakage due to the application of excessive traction and heat to relaxed hair. Negroid hair is particularly susceptible to damage due to its cross-sectional structure.

ture at the sites of the nodes, leading to patchy or diffuse alopecia.

Proximal trichorrhexis nodsa is common in those with typical Negroid hair. Repeated straightening by hot combing, relaxers or permanent waves is usually a feature of the history, compounded by physical damage from combing or brushing. Recovery may take between 2 and 4 years after cessation of these factors.

Distal trichorrhexis nodosa is seen mostly in whites and Orientals. The characteristic nodes appear on the distal few centimetres of hair, which is the older and therefore more weathered portion. The hair looks dull, uneven and dry and may be thinned and fragile.

Bubble hairs

Bubble hairs (Fig. 2.70) are characterized by the appearance of rows of bubbles within the hair shaft under the microscope. No obvious abnormality of the hair cuticle is present. The cause is excessive heat to the hair shaft, which causes intracortical water to expand. Hair dryers, which reach temperatures of 120–180 °C, are a significant cause. The hair may break due to cortical disruption.

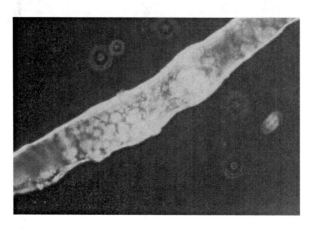

Fig. 2.70 Bubble hair caused by the boiling of water within the hair shaft due to overheating hair dryer on wet hair.

CASE STUDY

The full impact of weathering can be illustrated by the following case study.

This patient with naturally very curly, black hair worn to shoulder length (Fig. 2.71) has, clinically, dull, dry and brittle hair with obvious damage through repeated bleaching. There has been an episode of hair loss which the patient recognizes as hair breakage. This is the outcome of repeated bleaching with 60% peroxide accentuated by daily excessive use of a hair dryer.

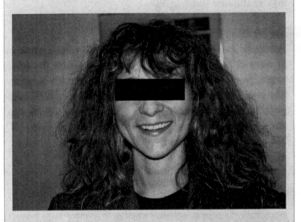

Fig. 2.71 Clinical appearance of hair severely weathered by repeated bleaching; the hair is friable and has lost its reflective qualities.

The hair is almost totally denuded of its coating and pliability and is exquisitely vulnerable to continuing damage.

A light microscopic examination (Fig. 2.72) reveals significant cortical disruption only 3 cm from the scalp.

The patient attributed the condition of her hair to childbirth and was unaware of the true nature of the problem. Cessation of bleaching and a reduction in blow-drying plus the use of mild shampoos and silicone-containing conditioners will significantly protect the existing hair, whilst continuing anagen growth proceeds to deliver 'normal' hair.

Continued on p. 77

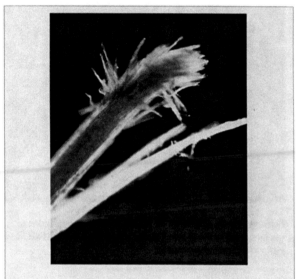

Fig. 2.72 Severe damage to the cortex on hair only 3 cm long.

Tangling and matting

Tangling of hair is very common, particularly when the hair is long, wet and regularly shampooed with strong detergents.

Severe matting of the hair may occur, particularly if the hair is weathered.

Long hair is susceptible to the uncommon but catastrophic physical phenomenon of felting, which results from the tangling by friction during washing (Fig. 2.73). This may occur when hair is washed while piled on top of the head (a method that should always be avoided) rather than as a backwash.

The phenomenon has been described as 'bird's nest hair'. Since severe felting is irreversible, the hair invariably has to be cut off.

MANAGEMENT OF WEATHERING

In general, the correct treatment for patients with severely weathered hair is aimed at minimizing further physical and chemical trauma.

In some cases professional cutting is a first step.

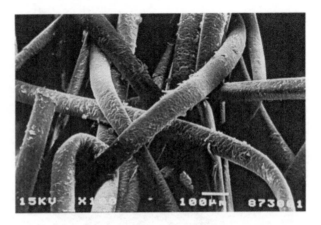

Fig. 2.73 'Bird's nest hair': the felting of the long hair is due to washing it while it was piled on the top of the head; the hair has a history of chemical treatment.

The role of modern cosmetic products

Only shampoos with a mild surfactant system tailored to the individual need should be used. These include variants for a range of processed hair.

Conditioners, which reduce further damage by preventing tangling or matting and by improving hydration and decreasing friction damage, are essential on a regular and even a daily basis. Silicone conditioning agents are useful specifically in preventing damage to the cuticle. They deposit on the cuticular edge and help to prevent ratchet interlocking with other hairs. This is essential where the inherent hydrophobic fatty acid layer has been stripped by chemical treatment.

Coarse hairbrushes should be avoided and wide-toothed combs should be used, particularly when the hair is wet, in order to minimize trauma.

Tightly drawn ponytails and tight braids should be avoided.

For long hair, it is important to shampoo in running water without piling the hair on the head.

The use of permanent waves, hair straighteners, relaxers, hair dyes, and treatment involving heat, such as hot combing, hot curlers and curling irons, should be restricted in all cases of hair fragility.

Congenital and hereditary shaft defects

IRREGULARITIES IN SHAPE

Twisting and coiling
These rare abnormalities may be associated with clinical fragility. They can be classified as defects:
• with overt hair fragility; or
• without clinical fragility.
Congenital or hereditary hair shaft defects occur in about 1 in every 10 000 births, and may be associated with clinical and cosmetic problems. The following examples of specific morphological defects, although uncommon, should be considered when assessing patients with brittle hair.

WITH OVERT HAIR FRAGILITY

Pili torti
In pili torti, the affected hair shaft is flattened and twisted on its own axis, usually through an angle of 180° with a range of 90–360° (Fig. 2.74). The affected hairs are usually found in the occipital and temporal regions. They are brittle, break easily and do not grow to a normal length, causing a patchy alopecia.

Pili torti is usually congenital but may be acquired, as in scarring alopecia.

The classic type of pili torti (Ronchese) is a diffuse abnormality usually found in childhood in association with thin, blond hair. It may occur alone or as part of an ectodermal dysplasia syndrome with widely spaced teeth and enamel hypoplasia, nail dystrophy, corneal opacities, keratosis pilaris and ichthyosis.

Menkes' syndrome, in which pili torti occurs in combination with excessive weathering, is a congenital defect in copper metabolism.

Corkscrew hair is a unique type of twisting in which many hairs are twisted in a double spiral. It occurs in association with widely spaced teeth and syndactyly of fingers and toes, and may be familial.

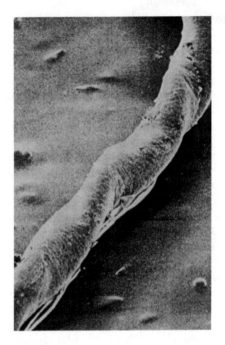

Fig. 2.74 Classical pili torti.

Management of pili torti. There is no recognized medical treatment for pili torti but the hair may grow longer if trauma from hair styling is minimized. In this respect the use of modern cosmetic hair care products is of enormous benefit. Regular conditioning is essential to prevent tangling and reduce friction in grooming.

Monilethrix

Monilethrix hair shafts show characteristic elliptical nodes with a beaded appearance, 0.7–1 mm apart, with intervening, tapered constrictions that are nonmedullated (Fig. 2.75).

The nodes occur at seemingly regular intervals and the intervening hair shaft is not twisted. The 'beading' may be obvious on clinical examination. Weathering may lead to a loss of cuticle cells over the nodes, which are exposed

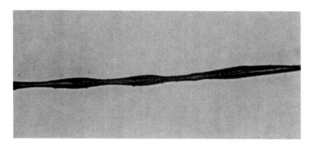

Fig. 2.75 Monilethrix may lead to hair breakage where trauma affects the exposed beads.

to maximal trauma. Hence the beaded hairs are extremely fragile and break off short, causing considerable hair loss.

Monilethrix usually appears in early childhood but can occur as late as the second decade of life.

There is no specific treatment for monilethrix but it may spontaneously disappear in adults. Oral etretinate has been reported to improve hair growth, as has topical minoxidil, despite the fact that the nodes persist.

Trichorrhexis invaginata (bamboo hair)

Trichorrhexis invaginata, or 'bamboo hair' presents as nodules on the hair shaft in which a ball-and-socket joint or bamboo-shaped node is formed (Fig. 2.76).

Clinically, multiple small nodules are seen along the shaft at irregular intervals. The hair is usually short, thin and friable. Bamboo hair occurs with ichthyosis, a scaly skin disorder, in Netherton's syndrome.

Trichomalacia

Trichomalacia, the term applied to damaged and twisted hair within the hair follicle, results from damage to the hair root during anagen. The best examples are seen in **trichotillomania**, in which a compulsive desire to pull out one's own hair becomes a damaging habit (Fig. 2.77). The condition, which is more common in females than in males, is relatively benign in young children but more severe and often indicative of underlying psychiatric disorders in older age groups. The diagnosis is usually made from the history and observation.

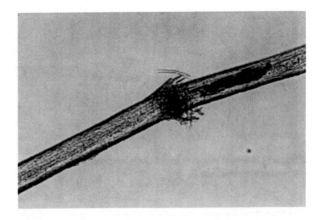

Fig. 2.76 'Bamboo hair' is associated with Netherton's syndrome, a rare disorder also characterized by ichthyosis linearis circumflexa. Clinically, sparse fragile hairs are seen.

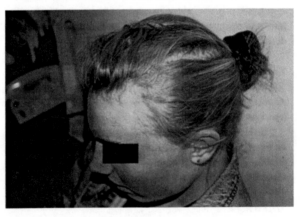

(a)

Fig. 2.77 Trichotillomania. (a) Hair loss at both temples. This patient self-diagnosed her condition; examination stress was a significant factor.

Hairs of different lengths are found in the areas of hair loss. The histological changes of trichotillomania and other forms of traction alopecia, such as hair weaves, are similar in that large numbers of catagen and telogen hairs may be accompanied by varying degrees of trichomalacia. Chronic traction alopecia along scalp hair margins, such as that

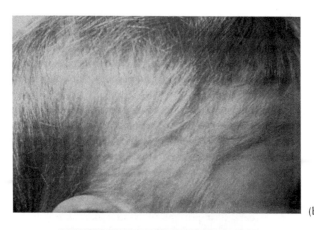

(b)

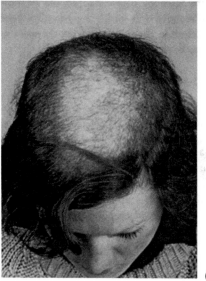

(c)

Fig. 2.77 *Continued* (b) Childhood type. (c) Severe. A key diagnostic factor is the clinical observation of growing hairs of different lengths.

caused by a tightly pulled ponytail, often causes permanent scarring of many hair follicles.

In the treatment of trichotillomania, the underlying emotional or psychosomatic problems must be addressed.

Pili annulati
Pili annulati, or ringed hairs, have characteristic alternating light and dark bands in the hair shafts, which give the hair a ringed or sandy appearance. The rings can be seen both clinically and under the light microscope, but are seen most readily in blond hair.

The abnormal bands have many cortical air-filled spaces, and the hairs are liable to fracture at these points. Obvious hair damage is uncommon in pili annulati, however; the condition can even impart an attractive appearance to the hair.

Treatment of fragile hair
Gentle care is important with all types of fragile hair. Constant brushing of the hair should be avoided, and it should be styled only with a wide-toothed comb or styling brush. Modern shampoos and conditioners are of prime importance for non-damaging hair care.

WITHOUT OVERT FRAGILITY

Longitudinal ridging and grooving
Longitudinal grooving is probably the single most common hair shaft irregularity (Fig. 2.78). It is frequently seen in normal hair and in many ectodermal dysplasias, and also in loose anagen hair syndrome. The latter occurs in young, usually blonde girls aged 2–5; anagen hairs with ruffled cuticles and no root sheaths are easily pulled from the scalp.

Hair grooving reflects a normal variation or a congenital abnormality of the hair shaft, and is not in itself a cause of increased hair fragility.

Infectious, physical and inflammatory causes of hair loss
The alopecia resulting from these conditions may be either temporary or permanent. It is usually of a focal (unifocal or multifocal) nature and commonly is associated with scalp inflammation.

Tinea capitis
Certain species of dermatophytes may cause **tinea capitis** (Fig. 2.79 (a)), which occurs mostly but not exclusively in

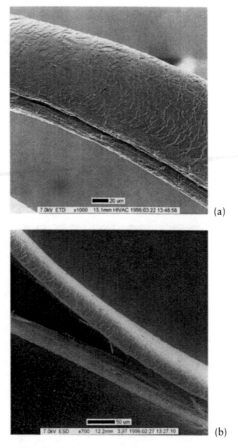

Fig. 2.78 Grooving of the hair is the most frequent irregularity. It is most common in Negroid hair.

prepubertal children. Around half the cases of tinea capitis in patients over the age of 20 occur in individuals over 60 years of age. Tinea capitis caused by *Microsporum* (Fig. 2.79 (b)) organisms is transmitted primarily from animals to humans, in whom there is frequently spontaneous resolution. *M. canis* (Fig. 2.79 (c)) is the organism most commonly involved.

Hair breakage associated with follicular inflammation accounts for the patchy loss.

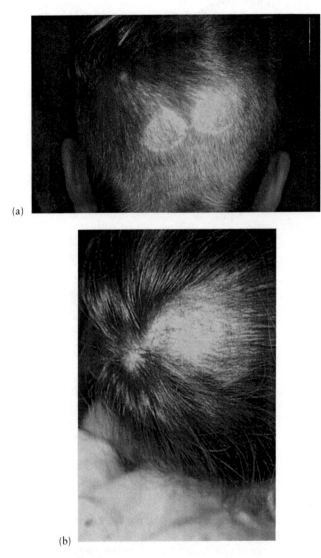

(a)

(b)

Fig. 2.79 Tinea capitis.

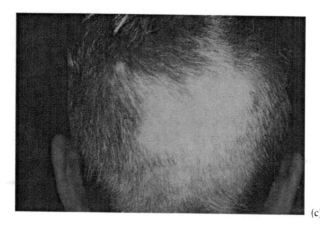

(c)

Fig. 2.79 *Continued.*

Tinea tonsurans is transmitted from person to person and is contagious: the infection can be passed by adults to successive generations of children by transfer of organisms from combs, brushes, caps and linens.

Favus

T. schoenleinii is occasionally seen in practice. Yellow, cup-shaped crusts develop around the hair to form a confluent mass of yellow crusting. Extensive patchy hair loss with scarring and atrophy may develop, and may become irreversible.

Oral antifungal treatment is necessary. In confirmed cases systemic treatment is indicated, ketoconazole or fluconazole being the drugs of choice.

Psoriasis

This condition can give rise to a degree of alopecia; see page 103.

Folliculitis decalvans

This is probably an abnormal host response to common bacteria. Lesions are those of chronic and overt pustulation leading to progressive scarring (Fig. 2.80). Patients should be investigated for underlying defects of the immune

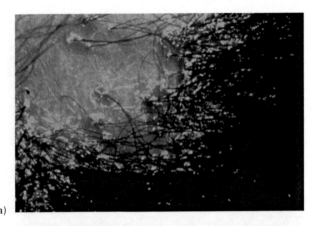

(a)

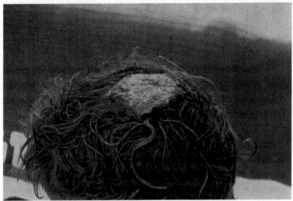

(b)

Fig. 2.80 (a) Folliculitis decalvans is associated with chronic and overt pustulation. (b) Kerion. This is the most serious form of ringworm due to *Trichophyton verrucosum* or *T. mentagrophytes*.

response. Antibiotics will suppress the disease but only whilst they are delivered.

These cases will almost certainly require expert help and any case where there is a suggestion of a scarring alopecia should be referred.

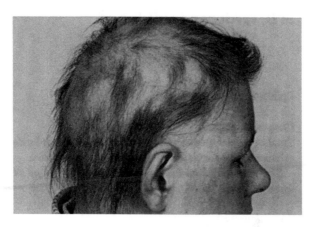

Fig. 2.81 The secondary stage of syphilis is not uncommonly seen, but recovers after treatment.

Syphilis

In the primary stage of syphilis, there is no scalp hair loss unless there is a primary lesion in the scalp. It is not uncommon in the secondary and tertiary stages, however.

Hair loss in secondary syphilis (Fig. 2.81) takes the form of irregular 'moth-eaten' areas of loss of hair scattered throughout the scalp, similar to patchy alopecia areata. The eyebrows may be shed and there may be a patchy alopecia in the beard and other hair-bearing areas of the body. A second presentation in secondary syphilis is a diffuse hair loss resembling that seen in telogen effluvium. Hair regrowth and decreased telogen counts can begin 4–6 weeks after starting treatment.

3: Disorders of childhood

Childhood alopecia

Congenital alopecia
Total or partial alopecia occurs either as an isolated defect or in association with a wide range of other anomalies.

Circumscribed alopecia is due to local aplasia of all skin layers or an epidermal naevus.

Total alopecia
This is an isolated defect (autosomal recessive) which may be dominant in families. Adult hair follicles are absent, though there may have been lanugo hair. Scalp hair is normal at birth but is shed up to the age of 6 months. Other body hair may be absent. Teeth and nails are normal, and the child is normal in other respects as well.

Hypotrichosis
Congenital hypotrichosis (autosomal dominant) may cause social problems. It is seldom severe. It may be a secondary feature to other syndromes. In these conditions the hair may be sparse and fragile, with monithelix and pili torti.

Certain rare neonatal conditions expressed as alopecia fall into the broad group of hypotrichoses. The group is a diagnostic mixture of cases with decreased follicular numbers, smaller follicles or fragile abnormal hairs.

Marie–Unna syndrome (Fig. 3.1) is a rare but distinctive autosomal dominant condition. Some patients are normal at birth, while others are bald. The hair is sparse until the age of three, when coarse, flattened twisted hair appears on the scalp. This is slowly lost at puberty around the scalp margins and on the vertex.

Epidermal naevi are usually hairless warty plaques.

Aplasia cutis, mimicking alopecia areata (AA) is occasion-

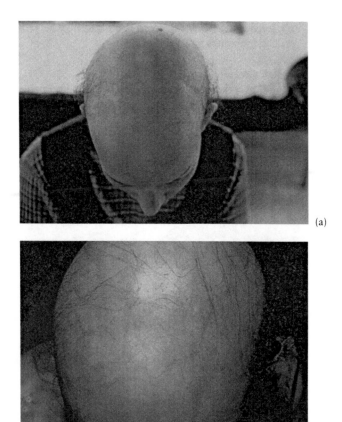

(a)

(b)

Fig. 3.1 Marie–Unna syndrome.

ally seen (Fig. 3.2). This is a congenital defect due to aplasia of all layers.

Pseudopelade may occur in infants in association with other hereditary syndromes (Conradi's syndrome).

Trichothiodystrophy
This is a disorder of sulphur metabolism. Various syndrome complexes have been described. Clinically there is brittle

hair, intellectual impairment and short stature. The hair is weak and weathers poorly (see Fig. 2.65).

Physiological alopecia
Children may develop apparent hair loss due to the development of mosaic patterns or an area of normal telogen loss at about 12 weeks of age (see Fig. 1.2, p. 2). This is widely and wrongly attributed to friction.

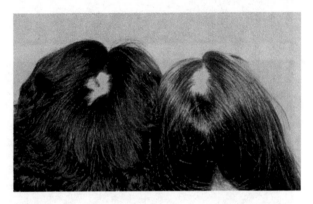

Fig. 3.2 Aplasia cutis may mimic AA.

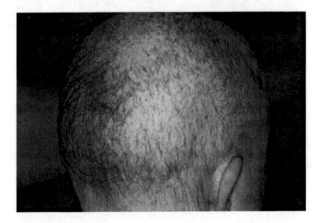

Fig. 3.3 Monilethrix.

Other childhood alopecias

Alopecia areata and **trichotillomania** (see pages 60 and 81) are seen in children.

Monilethrix occurs in childhood, the hair is typically beaded and tends to breakage.

In addition there is a condition, usually found in fair-haired girls, called **loose anagen syndrome** in which the hair is easily and painlessly pulled out of the scalp. It is due to a weakness in the hair root. It may improve with age.

For further reading, see RSM ICSS (1996) *The hairshaft — aesthetics, disease and damage.*

Unruly hair in children

Children may often be observed with unruly or uncombable hair (Fig. 3.4).

Unruly hair with no obvious hair shaft abnormality is sometimes seen in the newborn, but spontaneously disappears within 12–18 months of birth. It may occur in normal infants, but is in some cases associated with Down's syndrome or other congenital or hereditary defects.

So-called **congenital unruly hair** associated with a hair shaft structural abnormality arises after 3 months of age.

The condition of non-fragile, unruly hair includes all

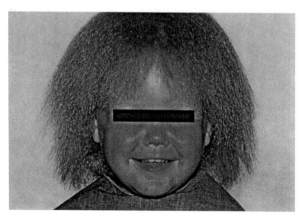

Fig. 3.4 Cheveux incoiffables is associated with an irregularity of the hair shaft.

forms of woolly hair and uncombable hair (*cheveux incoif-fables*, Fig. 3.4).

Several possible causes of fragile unruly hair, which may include all forms of pili torti, have been discussed above.

Uncombable hair
Uncombable hair syndrome is characterized by hair shafts that are mainly triangular or kidney-shaped in cross-section (Fig. 3.5) and have a longitudinal groove. The entire hair shaft is involved, but the cuticle is intact and twists or bends are unusual.

Uncombable hair syndrome is sometimes noticed in young infants, but may not appear until as late as age 12. It is usually seen by the time the child is 3 years old and may persist for life, although it has been known for spontaneous improvement to occur in later childhood.

The hairs do not usually weather significantly. The hair usually has a characteristic silvery-blond colour, but can be straw-coloured. It sticks out from the scalp, is disorderly and cannot be combed flat.

Straight hair naevus has been suggested as a focal naevoid form of uncombable hair syndrome.

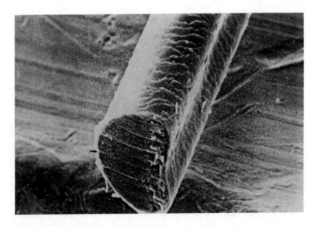

Fig. 3.5 EMG of cheveux incoiffables showing characteristic kidney-shaped cross-section.

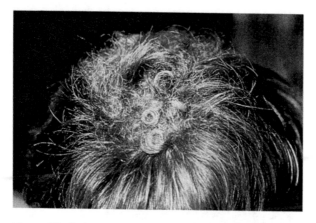

Fig. 3.6 Woolly hair naevus.

Woolly hair

'Woolly' hair, which resembles Negroid hair, is seen in white Caucasoids.

Woolly hair is unruly and difficult to style because it does not lie flat or form normal locks (Fig. 3.6). The hair is tightly coiled, curled or kinked, and individual hairs are usually ovoid rather than round. Their shaft diameter is small. Some degree of weathering is common, but fragility is unusual.

Trichonodosis

In trichonodosis (knotted hair), a single, or sometimes a double, knot occurs in the hair shaft (Fig. 3.7). Slack knots, often in considerable numbers, may be produced by friction on pillows and by various cosmetic procedures. Short, curly hair of both the Negroid and the Caucasoid type is particularly susceptible to knotting. Straight hair is much less likely to be affected.

Combing may tighten the knots. It may even pull out anagen hair, and can cause a fracture of the hair shaft at the site of the knot.

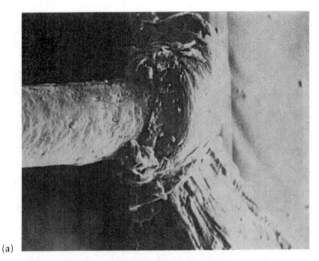

(a)

(b)

Fig. 3.7 Short curly hair, particularly Negroid hair, is susceptible to knotting.

Scalp disorders

Seborrhoeic dermatitis

This condition develops during the first few weeks or months or life. It is uncertain whether this is the same condition as the adult form.

Grey, greasy crusts form on the scalp in the first few weeks or months of life, and erythema may develop in skin folds. It may be associated with atopy, but is not always so.

It resolves spontaneously, and parents should be reassured.

4: Extraneous matter

Patients may present with various kinds of material adhering to the hair or the scalp. Potential causes include the following:
- fungi;
- tinea capitis;
- piedra;
- bacteria;
- trichomycosis axillaris;
- pediculosis;
- nits (Figs 4.1 & 4.2);
- perpilar casts;
- pseudonits;
- deposits; and
- spray lacquer, paint, glue.

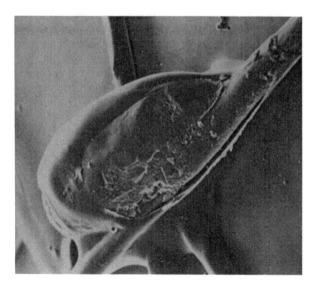

Fig. 4.1 Nits only hatch close to the scalp; they do not affect adult males.

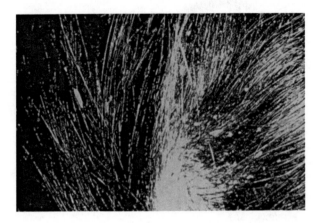

Fig. 4.2 Nits in black hair.

Hair shaft deposits

Deposits of extraneous material from many sources can adhere to hair shafts. Usually these particles are not distributed throughout the scalp but are localized to areas of contact.

The diagnosis can usually be made by history and clinical examination. Evaluation under the microscope will establish that the extraneous matter is not an inherent part of the hair shaft.

5: Disorders of the scalp

Scalp problems are not infrequently encountered in primary practice. Most are relatively benign but some may be chronic, and also cosmetically embarrassing for the patient.

Dandruff

Dandruff is a near-physiological scaling of the scalp, which may or may not be associated with skin greasiness (seborrhoea). It is alternatively known as **pityriasis simplex** or **furfuracea**.

Dandruff is an affliction particularly of adolescence and adult life and is relatively rare and mild in children. Its peak incidence and severity are reached at the age of about 20 years; by this age, some 50% of white Caucasians have been affected to some degree. It usually clears spontaneously during the fifth or sixth decade, though it may (rarely) persist in old age.

The age of incidence and the fact that it is most common in males suggests that an androgenic influence is at work, and the level of sebaceous activity may be a factor. Gross seborrhoea may occur without dandruff, however, and commonly severe dandruff may be present without any excessive sebaceous activity being clinically apparent.

The role of *Malassezia furfur* is still disputed in terms of whether it is the primary (determining) factor or whether it is one of the links in the chain of events that lead to dandruff. It is clear that *M. furfur* populations significantly increase in cases of dandruff, and also that reducing this population decreases the scaling.

Clinical features

Dandruff has the clinical feature of an accumulation of small white or grey scales on the surface of the scalp, either in localized patches or more diffusely (Fig. 5.1). After removal with an effective shampoo the scales form again within 4–7 days.

There are long- and short-term variations in its severity

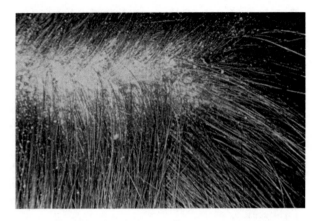

Fig. 5.1 Dandruff scales will reform within a few days of removal.

and in the ease with which the scales become detached and show prominently on the hair, scalp and shoulders.

In those subjects whose scalp becomes greasy at or after puberty, the seborrhoea binds the scale in a greasy 'paste' and it is no longer shed, but accumulates in small adherent mounds, the so-called **pityriasis steatoides**. The development of clinically evident inflammatory changes in such individuals may lead to seborrhoeic dermatitis.

Pruritus is not a feature of simple pityriasis. It is very much more common when inflammatory changes develop in seborrhoeic scalps. Acne necrotica, which may be intensely irritating, also can complicate pityriasis.

DIFFERENTIAL DIAGNOSIS
In a young child, the presence of more than very mild pityriasis throws doubt on the diagnosis. Extreme and persistent scale, even though it may lack the characteristic features of psoriasis, is always suspect, particularly if there is a family history of this disease. Widespread scaling, sometimes with scarring, may occur in some forms of ichthyosis. At any age, if pruritus is troublesome, pediculosis must be carefully excluded.

Small areas of scaling with dull broken hair shafts are typical of *Microsporon* ringworms. Localized scaling in children is therefore an indication for examination of the scalp under Wood's light, and of the broken hairs under the microscope. A nervous hair-pulling tic may result in twisted and broken hairs of normal texture in a patch of postinflammatory scaling.

Profuse sticky silvery scale that mats the hairs together should suggest **pityriasis amiantacea** (see below).

TREATMENT

Pityriasis in its milder forms is a physiological process. The object of treatment is to control it at the lowest possible cost and inconvenience to the patient, appreciating that any procedure found to be effective will need to be repeated at regular intervals.

Traditionally, particularly where seborrhoea was associated, a tar preparation was used and washed out after a few hours with shampoo. This treatment, which has to be repeated at intervals, is cosmetically unacceptable to many nowadays.

Shampoos containing agents able to reduce the yeast population are generally very easy to use in the cosmetic sense and have demonstrated significant results. Other products used to reduce dandruff contain keratolytic agents, mostly in pharmaceutical preparation; these are able to disrupt and peel away cells of the horny layer of the skin, but this does lead to a further reduction in the thickness of the horny layer.

Other treatments such as selenium sulphide have been shown to reduce epidermal turnover; they are useful for some patients, but fail inexplicably in others.

Antipityrosporum therapy with imidazole compounds such as ketoconazole has some anti-inflammatory and antiandrogenic effects, which may be important.

Zinc pyrithione in a retail shampoo has been shown to be as effective as OTC and RX treatments.

Pityriasis amiantacea (asbestos-like scale)

This term describes a scalp reaction, often idiopathic, with asbestos-like scales. It may occur at any age, but the average lies between 5 and 40. It may be associated with psoriasis.

The characteristic feature is masses of sticky silvery scales adhering to the scalp in layers. The scalp may be red and moist. The condition is usually confined to a small area of the scalp but occasionally it is extensive. Most patients observe some hair loss in areas of severe scaling.

Treatment consists of shampooing with a tar-based or imidazole preparation, and where necessary the application of topical antibiotics and/or steroids.

Seborrhoea

A typical patient produces sebum in quantities that he or she regards as excessive, and complains of excessive greasiness and unmanageable hair. There is an association with hirsutism, which may indicate increased androgen activity. The menstrual history is important and if abnormal should be investigated.

Proprietary cosmetic shampoos are adequate for most of the patients in whom there is no indication for systemic treatment.

Seborrhoeic dermatitis

The cause of this condition is unknown. It can occur in infants when sebaceous activity is established. Histologically it has features of chronic eczema and psoriasis (Fig. 5.2).

Greasy scales with exudate form crusts and the scalp is

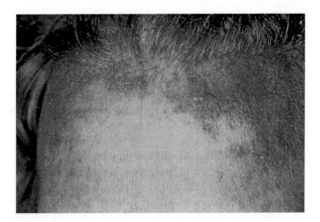

Fig. 5.2 Seborrhoeic dermatitis has features of both chronic eczema and psoriasis.

erythematous and moist. The eyebrows and nasolabial folds are often involved and the scalp may ultimately be affected, with extensive dermatitis beyond the frontal margin. Beards may increase the incidence on the face, and the post auricular area may become affected too.

Secondary infection may occur with pustules.

TREATMENT

Corticosteroid lotion is useful. The regular use of shampoos with antifungal activity is important.

Secondary infection should be aggressively treated with systemic antibiotics.

Psoriasis

Psoriasis is a genetically determined disorder affecting 1.5–2% of the population of northwest Europe. The mean age of onset is in the third decade of life. Diagnosis is by examination for other lesions in association with family history.

The scalp is frequently involved and the condition typically presents as a palpable bright pink plaque covered in silvery scale (Fig. 5.3) (in children this may be less distinctive). In a severe case there may be a solid cap extending beyond the hair margin. There may be patchy or diffuse scaling, or alternatively thick asbestos like scales. Some

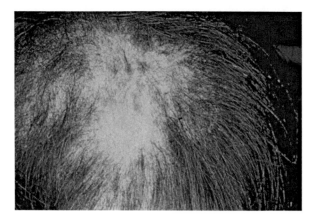

Fig. 5.3 The silvery scales typical of psoriasis.

increased shedding of telogen hairs is common in psoriasis plaques, but extensive hair loss occurs only in the erythrodermic forms.

Treatment consists of the use of tar-based shampoos; salicylic acid may be useful in combination with these. Corticosteroid scalp lotions may be helpful. The patient must be counselled on the need for daily compliance.

Index

Index

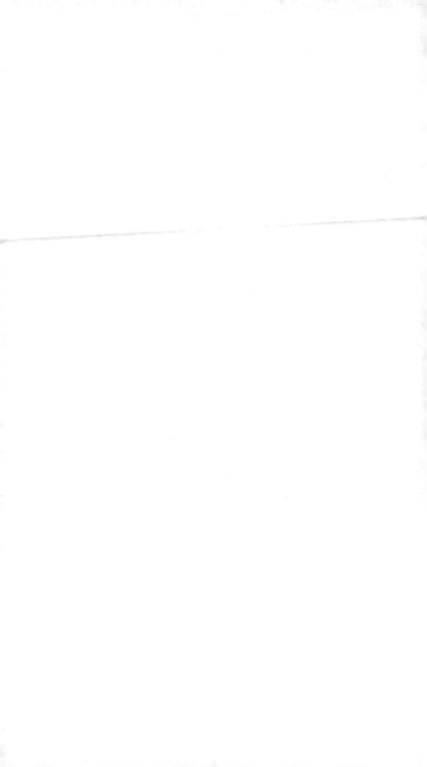

Lightning Source UK Ltd.
Milton Keynes UK
UKOW04f0606130614

233304UK00001B/2/P